The Institute of Biology's
Studies in Biology no. 28

The Biology
of Respiration

by Christopher Bryant M.Sc., Ph.D.(Lond)

Senior Lecturer in Zoology
Australian National University
Canberra

Edward Arnold

First published 1971
by Edward Arnold (Publishers) Limited,
41 Maddox Street,
London, W1R 0AN

Boards edition ISBN: 0 7131 2307 9
Paper edition ISBN: 0 7131 2308 7

305217

Printed in Great Britain by
William Clowes and Sons Ltd, London, Beccles and Colchester

General Preface to the Series

It is no longer possible for one textbook to cover the whole field of Biology and to remain sufficiently up to date. At the same time students at school, and indeed those in their first year at universities, must be contemporary in their biological outlook and know where the most important developments are taking place.

The Biological Education Committee, set up jointly by the Royal Society and the Institute of Biology, is sponsoring, therefore, the production of a series of booklets dealing with limited biological topics in which recent progress has been most rapid and important.

A feature of the series is that the booklets indicate as clearly as possible the methods that have been employed in elucidating the problems with which they deal. Wherever appropriate there are suggestions for practical work for the student. To ensure that each booklet is kept up to date, comments and questions about the contents may be sent to the author or the Institute.

1971

Institute of Biology
41 Queen's Gate
London, S.W.7

Preface

The urge to write this book derives from the feeling that there is a balance to be redressed. A large proportion of biochemists devote their time to mammals and micro-organisms, forgetting, for example, that mammals comprise only a single Class in a rather small Phylum, the Chordata. Many of these biochemists lavish attention on small systems, isolated *in vitro*, without paying too much attention to the roles of such systems *in vivo*. I do not under-rate such work; these approaches are essential, of proven value—and inevitable, because Man is, by definition, anthropocentric. His first thought is 'how does this affect *me?*', and medical research, in particular, has little time to speculate on the functions of enzymes in water snails—unless those snails happen to harbour a parasite which is injurious to man.

The present book is written for *biologists*, as distinct from biochemists, botanists and zoologists. If the chemist finds that the treatment of his concepts is less rigorous than he would like, or the zoologist finds that assumptions about some animals are rather naive, I ask them to forgive me and consider the main theme—which is that all life is the proper study of the biologist.

This booklet is designed to follow on from an earlier book in this series—Geoffrey R. Barker's *Understanding the Chemistry of the Cell*. Concepts developed there are fundamental to the understanding of the present work.

Canberra, 1971

C.B.

Contents

Preface   iii

1   Ecology and Respiration   1

2   Respiration and Electron Transport   5
    2.1   Methods for studying respiration   5
    2.2   Oxidation and electron transfer   11
    2.3   The mitochondrion   14
    2.4   Electron transport in biological systems   16

3   Oxidative Phosphorylation   24
    3.1   Introduction   24
    3.2   History   25
    3.3   Substrate-linked phosphorylation   28
    3.4   Respiratory chain phosphorylation   29

4   Doing Without Oxygen   36
    4.1   Aerobiosis and anaerobiosis   36
    4.2   The oxygen debt   38
    4.3   Diving animals   42
    4.4   Intermediate cases   44
    4.5   Hibernation   44
    4.6   Diapause   46

5   A Long-term Solution—Intestinal Parasites   50
    5.1   Introduction   50
    5.2   Metabolic pathways in parasites   51
    5.3   Electron transport in parasites   53
    5.4   The switch mechanism   55

6   Conclusions   57

Further Reading   60

Ecology and Respiration 1

The relationship between the environment of an animal and its respiratory metabolism is a very intimate one which has been often neglected by biochemists. An animal is fitted to its environment, and the fitness is manifested at the cellular level as well as at the level of the whole animal; unfortunately, the finer details tend to be overlooked. Considerable attention has been paid in the literature to physiological mechanisms underlying the adaptation of an animal to its ecological niche, but much less to the way in which biochemical mechanisms, in turn, provide the foundation which makes this adaptation possible.

It is important that the serious student of biology should realize early that all life is not described by the common laboratory animals and Man, and that he should also realize the dangers of considering animals apart from their environments. The environment makes demands on the organism; together, environment and organism make a unit which should ideally be studied as a unit. It is this concept that makes ecology the most important of today's biological sciences.

Environments which are different in many ways may yet have one or more important features in common which result in similar adaptations in the animals which occupy them. It is therefore necessary that great care should be taken to avoid the danger of postulating relationships between groups of animals on the basis of biochemical similarities. Such similarities may be the result of a common need, rather than a common ancestor. As an example, it proved to be erroneous to erect a hypothesis for the origin of vertebrates on a single biochemical system. It was suggested that echinoderm ancestors were related to ancestral vertebrates, because, amongst other things, both groups possessed creatine phosphate as an energy store. Invertebrates were thought to be the exclusive possessors of arginine phosphate. Unfortunately for this hypothesis, as larger numbers of groups were studied, echinoderms and invertebrates generally were found to possess both phosphagens. The distribution of phosphagens in the animal kingdom is based at least as much on the need for an energy store, whatever the components of the mechanism that produces it, as on an evolutionary relationship.

The bottom of a muddy pond is usually rich in organic matter and poor in oxygen. Occupation of environments like this may result in the appearance in organisms of adaptations which resemble those found in organisms from other oxygen deficient environments. For example, there are common features in the cellular respiration of free-living flatworms from the pond, and the respiration of worms parasitic in the small intestine of the sheep. They may indeed be due to a relationship, for the flatworm and the parasite are usually included in the same phylum, and the worms' respective successes in the ditch or in the gut may be because their ancestors possessed respiratory adaptations which permitted them to exploit oxygen-poor environments. Or it may be that the animals are unrelated, and that they responded in a similar way to a similar challenge.

Another point to be considered is the conservative nature of life. Similar answers may be arrived at even where problems are only loosely connected. The occurrence of haemoglobin in such widely diverse forms as vertebrates, molluscs, insect larvae and intestinal parasites merely reflects the usefulness of a sub-group of haemoproteins in transactions which involve the transport and storage of small molecules like oxygen.

An important property of life is that it runs counter to the physical processes of the universe. The universe is running down, moving from a highly ordered state to a completely disordered one. On the other hand, life is characterized by its high degree of order which is maintained in the face of events which tend to break it down. The continued existence of life is therefore dependent on a continuous supply of energy to repair the depredations caused by the environment. Although its ultimate origin is solar radiation, in animals energy is made available during the processes of respiration; it is not surprising that a system which fulfils such a basic requirement arose early in evolution and has been largely resistant to innovation. It must have arisen early and it must have been perfected early; subsequent modification has hardly been required.

The term respiration includes a variety of activities, from the metabolic pathways which enable the accomplishment of the capture of chemical energy, to the physiological and behavioural mechanisms which enable the organism to sample a portion of its environment, and extract from it oxygen which may enter solution in the body fluids and ultimately become available to the individual cells. It is at the latter levels that the greatest variability is encountered, because the body surface of the organism, whether an elephant or *Amoeba*, makes intimate contact with the outer world. External surfaces and forms are therefore the most plastic of structures. They interact with, and are moulded by the environment, and their natures are dictated by the necessity for keeping the environment at bay. Elephant's hide and *Amoeba* membranes are two ways of achieving this. The surfaces are supportive, helping to maintain the integrity of the organisms, but they also form selective barriers which oxygen and other substances must somehow cross.

Now, as environments are variable, it is not at all surprising to find that there are many mechanisms for taking what is required of them. In *Amoeba*, diffusion is sufficient to transport oxygen from the environment to all parts of the organism. As it is an aquatic animal, it needs no elaborate devices for getting the oxygen into solution; oxygen arrives in that condition at the body surface, which is an advantage shared by most aquatic organisms, whether freshwater or marine.

As the size of the organism increases, skeletal and defensive requirements may result in most of the body becoming enclosed in armour of various sorts. Under these circumstances, a specialized respiratory surface develops, where the soft parts are directly exposed to the environment. Such a surface may be a vastly elaborated epithelium hidden under a carapace, as in the crayfish, or merely those parts which are exposed as they perform another function. An example is the tube foot of the sea-urchin. Increase in size also means that diffusion is no longer a suitable vehicle for the transport of oxygen and other substances throughout the animal. Some form of activated transport or circulatory system is necessary.

The need to maintain a relatively vulnerable surface for gaseous exchange renders the terrestrial organism more vulnerable than it might otherwise be. A moist membrane is required, so that oxygen arriving at its surface film can go into solution and pass across it; yet water loss must also be controlled. Considerable evaporation of water occurs through the tracheae of insects and lungs of vertebrates, and perpetuates their dependence on a source of external water, either free or with the diet. Many organisms living in deserts apparently survive on water generated during metabolic processes. It is clear that those functions which are at the mercy of the environment are as variable as external conditions.

Once inside the animal, however, it is a different story. All organisms possess the property of homoeostasis. In the face of a universe in which the degree of disorder is continually increasing, they seek to maintain themselves, to increase and grow. In the long run they lose the battle; probably all organisms are mortal. During their lifetimes, however, they endeavour to maintain internal conditions as steady as possible to provide the most favourable conditions for the continuance of life.

Over long periods there is evolutionary change. It should not be thought of as a failure of homoeostasis, but rather as a homoeostatic compromise under new conditions of environment. The result is the innate conservativeness of the living organism, a resistance to the change which still occurs, slowly but inexorably, over epochs; a resistance during which the basic cellular processes and the cellular environment change very little. The genetic machinery of an organism determines whether it will be a man or a mouse, but whether man or mouse, the principles upon which the machine works and the components which comprise it are similar. It is the *order* which is different. The fundamental needs for the survival of man or mouse are the same, and their metabolic machineries show even greater similarities, because in both animals, they do the same job.

This is a statement of the unifying principle of biochemistry. All organisms are alike, for there are only a limited number of ways of carrying out a given process efficiently, and the most efficient of these tends to be selected by all organisms. Animals resemble one another more nearly than they resemble plants, but a visitor to this planet would not hesitate to classify plants and animals under the same heading. Apart from a few special functions, differences are in the details of general processes. For example, the metabolic pathway for the fixation of carbon dioxide by green plants during photosynthesis shows resemblances to a pathway which occurs in mammalian liver. But plants convert the carbon dioxide to sugars, whereas animals use the path in reverse for the degradation of sugars to carbon dioxide and a number of other important metabolites. Bacteria show greater differences from animals and plants, but even in these organisms, metabolic processes are similar to those of the higher organisms. They may have a few extra properties which animals, for example, do not possess, but the converse is equally true. In the last analysis, even their genetic codes are similar, which is reflected in the fact that much research in this area is carried out on micro-organisms.

It is clear, therefore, that where there are differences, they are the result of a different way of life, of the occupation of a different ecological niche. Obviously, an autotrophe like grass will need a different set of enzymes from the heterotrophic cow that feeds on it, but both grass and cow live in an environment rich in oxygen. Organisms are metabolic opportunists and tend to use whatever is in plentiful supply, if it can be used. Cellular respiration in grass and the cow therefore converges at the point at which oxygen is essential.

Where differences occur in such a fundamental process as respiration, it is obviously important to try to find out why. In the following pages, the extent of the effect of the environment, as far as is known, will be examined, using examples drawn from the animal kingdom. Of especial interest are those modifications which occur in animals occupying environments which are deficient in oxygen, as do many intestinal parasites, or which cut themselves off, either physically or physiologically, from the oxygen supply. It must be emphasized that it is an area which is still fraught with problems, and there are many gaps in our knowledge.

There are short term solutions to the problems of survival without oxygen. Even active mammals have to cope with a relative or effective shortage of oxygen for short periods. One example is a man sprinting a hundred yards; a more interesting example is the sounding of the whale, which may stay submerged for hours at a time. They both illustrate how the animal frees itself from the constraints imposed on it by the environment, and where a basic process has undergone modification in response to environmental demands. Such modifications contribute materially to the success of the organism by opening up to it hitherto unexploited evolutionary niches.

It is the purpose of this book to attempt to determine where differences occur in the fundamental biochemical process of respiration. If changes do occur in such a basically stable metabolic system, then it is important to try to find the cause of the departure from the very successful and hence very conservative pattern. It is important, not only from the point of view of the intrinsic interest of the exercise, but from the point of view of understanding the animal and its relationship to its environment.

Respiration and Electron Transport 2

2.1 Methods for studying respiration

The earliest investigations into respiration were undertaken without any complicated equipment, although the experiments by which Lavoisier established that animals need oxygen would require a measure of ingenuity to duplicate even today. These and later studies all involved the enclosure of living material in air-tight vessels. Subsequent workers attached liquid-filled tubes called manometers. The change of the level of the liquid in a manometer gives a measure of the amount of oxygen which has been taken up. These devices were only possible if they possessed traps containing an alkali, which could absorb any carbon dioxide evolved. During aerobic respiration, the volume of carbon dioxide given out is close to the volume of oxygen utilized; when carbohydrates are being oxidized, the ratio is exactly 1. In the absence of a trap, therefore, there will be no volume change.

This approach culminated in the development by Otto Warburg of the famous respirometer, which is surely to be found lurking in every biochemical laboratory in the world. The Warburg apparatus is a constant volume device; that is, it is used to determine differences in volumes by measuring the drop in pressure which occurs when oxygen is used up in an enclosed flask. If the pressure drops, the true volume of gas inside the flask is, when corrected to normal temperature and pressure, obviously smaller. It can also be used to measure gas output. A modern Warburg apparatus possesses a mechanism for shaking the flasks in which the live material is placed, in order to ensure that the suspension medium remains fully saturated with respect to oxygen. It has a thermostatically controlled bath to maintain the temperature of the experimental material, and a thermobarometer which allows the experimenter to compensate for minor changes in temperature and fluctuations in pressure which would otherwise introduce errors into measurements. The manometers are fixed and the flasks are removable, and there is provision for replacing the atmosphere in the flasks with other gases. The most modern versions of the apparatus give the corrected volume of the gas change on a digital readout.

There are also constant pressure respirometers, which measure oxygen uptake directly as change in volume, but the Warburg apparatus has found greater application. It is suitable for whole animal work, if the animals are small enough, as well as for measuring the respiration of cellular and subcellular suspensions. For larger animals, say about the size of a rat, the Barcroft respirometer is often used, but the principles involved and the problems encountered are not dissimilar. In the last few years, increasing use has been made of the oxygen electrode for measuring oxygen uptake.

It is more sensitive than the manometric devices, and less easy to handle, but it is more accurate. An example of its use is given in Chapter 3.

The pioneer workers rightly considered that the interpretation of results obtained from the whole animal was too difficult to give a clear picture of the processes involved in respiration. They therefore had recourse to the use of excised tissues (liver, kidney and minced pigeon breast muscle were favourites). The tissues were employed either whole, which was of limited usefulness because of the failure of oxygen to penetrate rapidly throughout, or they were broken up in various ways. The different types of preparations included slices cut very thin; breis, in which the tissue was chopped into very small pieces; minces, and homogenates.

A whole sub-science has built up around the preparation of homogenates and the separation of sub-cellular particles from them. In carefully prepared homogenates, the cell membrane is ruptured, spilling out the contents of the cell unharmed. It was suspected as early as 1914 that one of the cell inclusions, the mitochondrion, was somehow implicated in respiration. The first efforts to isolate mitochondria for further study were those of Bensley, in the 1930's, and although he only achieved a partial success, it represented a great advance over previous work. Bensley was inhibited by lack of both the proper suspension medium and an adequate centrifuge. It was not until 1948 that Hogeboom, Schneider and Palade reported on the excellence of sucrose solutions for this purpose and the use of the technique of differential centrifugation for the preparation of intact mitochondria. Today, any manual of biochemistry will give the simple instructions which will enable anyone with access to a reasonable centrifuge to prepare a sample of mitochondria, suitable for all ordinary purposes, from rat liver.

In recent years, however, the need has arisen for absolutely pure preparations so that the worker can more easily distinguish between the respiratory and ancillary functions of the mitochondrion. This has led to a close scrutiny of all stages of preparation. The first step is the removal of the tissue to be investigated from the animal. Speed is essential as irreversible changes occur very soon after death. Experienced workers can remove rat liver, for example, and cool it in the appropriate medium (usually isotonic sucrose) within thirty seconds of killing. It is of paramount importance that the tissue be cooled to between $0°$ and $4°C$ as quickly as possible, to slow down any enzyme reactions which may contribute to the breakdown of the system under investigation. In some cases, even more rapid cooling is essential, and there are experiments described in the literature in which the whole rat is dunked in liquid nitrogen immediately after killing, in order to obtain an almost instantaneous cooling of the brain.

Having obtained the tissue and cooled and washed it in an appropriate medium, it is necessary next to homogenize it. A variety of tools have been used for this stage. One thing has to be borne in mind, however; the frictional heat generated by the homogenizer must not be allowed to warm the homogenate up, as damage may occur. Too vigorous homogenization may also denature the proteins. A commonly used homogenizer is the ordinary kitchen blender, or modifications of it. It is very useful for large quantities of material, but types which can process less than 1 ml are also available. Blenders such as these, however, are often too rough, and the shear forces

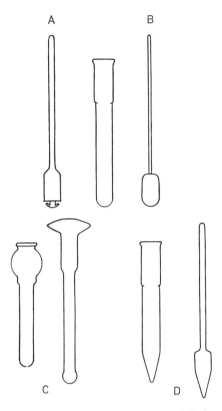

Fig. 2–1 Types of pestle homogenizers. A, B and D have pestles which just fit in the barrels. They are rotated by an overhead motor, while the barrel is moved slowly up and down. Type A is especially useful for tough, fibrous material as it is equipped with small stainless steel blades. Type C is most useful for soft tissues. The shear forces generated around the equator of the ball-ended pestle when it is pushed up and down are sufficient to rupture the cells.

generated by the blades may rupture the sub-cellular particle as well as the cell envelope. More frequently used are the pestle homogenizers of various types, which may be operated by hand or driven by a small electric motor (Fig. 2–1). Other common methods employed are sonic disruption, and rapid vibration in a vessel containing very small glass beads. With these two methods, there are greater problems associated with overheating. This list does not claim to be exhaustive; there are many other techniques not included here for reasons of space.

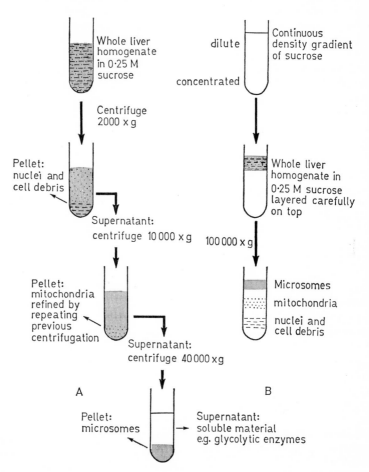

Fig. 2-2   Diagram illustrating the differences between differential (A) and density gradient centrifugation (B).

Once the homogenate has been obtained in the correct suspension medium, the required particle must be separated. Separation processes have been simplified in recent years by the development of superior centrifuges, some of which are capable of achieving centrifugal forces in excess of 200 000 times the force of gravity (g). There are two fundamental techniques, either of which results in the production of a satisfactory pre-paration of mitochondria, and other sub-cellular fractions.

The first technique is that of differential centrifugation, in which use is made of the fact that particles in the different fractions are of different sizes. Mitchondria are larger and heavier than microsomes, for example, and will sediment at a greater rate in a constant centrifugal field. Thus, a preliminary centrifugation at low speeds is employed to remove the large chunks of cell debris. The material which has remained in suspension after this treatment consists entirely of particles which are smaller than whole cells, and is called the supernatant. In the next run, the supernatant is centrifuged at about $10\ 000 \times g$, whereupon the mitochondria sediment under the increased centrifugal force. The supernatant from this spin will yield microsomes and other particles if desired. The mitochondrial pellet is usually washed several times by repeating the spin at $10\ 000 \times g$ before use.

An alternative technique is that of density gradient centrifugation. In this case, the homogenate is layered carefully on the top of the suspension medium in the centrifuge tube. The concentration of the medium in the tube has been carefully adjusted so that it forms a gradient in which it is highly concentrated at the bottom, and relatively dilute at the top. When it is subjected to high centrifugal force, the density gradient does not alter, but the elements from the homogenate will travel down the gradient until they reach the levels at which their own densities and that of the medium are equal. There will then be no further progress. When the centrifuge is stopped, the tube is carefully removed and the appropriate layer withdrawn by means of a hypodermic syringe.

Many of the techniques and pieces of apparatus mentioned in this section are exceedingly complex. However, even with the limited facilities available to them, the early workers provided a large amount of important data. Until the end of the 1930's, all of this information was derived from nothing more refined than a crude homogenate. Especially important were the remarkable studies of Otto Warburg; another worker who contributed much in this period was Thunberg. As an example of the sort of information that could be gained using quite unsophisticated apparatus, we can consider some of the experiments in which 'redox' dyes were used. The term 'redox potential' is a convenient contraction of oxidation-reduction potential. It is a quantitative measure of the readiness of a molecule to donate or accept electrons in oxidative or reductive reactions. The standard to which redox potentials are referred is the hydrogen electrode, where the following reaction takes place.

$$\tfrac{1}{2}H_2 \longrightarrow H^+ + e^-$$

The potential of this system is taken to be zero in a solution containing unit activity of hydrogen ions in equilibrium with hydrogen gas at a pressure of one atmosphere. Those systems which have a greater tendency to

donate electrons (reduction potentials) are assigned negative potentials
according to the recommendation of the International Union of Pure and
Applied Chemistry.

In the sense in which it is used here, the term 'redox dye' refers to dyes
which may donate or accept electrons in oxidation or reduction systems.
Thunberg developed a simple tube with a hollow, curved stopper and a
side-arm (Fig. 2–3). The tube could thus be completely evacuated, or its

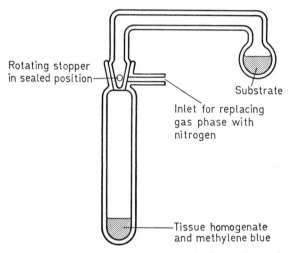

Fig. 2–3   Illustration of a simple experiment which may be performed with
a Thunberg tube. When the substrate, tissue homogenate and methylene
blue are mixed in an oxygen free system, the dye rapidly decolourizes.

atmosphere replaced with nitrogen or other gases. One of the redox dyes
he used was methylene blue, which acts as a sort of respiratory indicator.
When the dye is in the oxidized condition (its more usual state) it is a deep
blue. When it is reduced, it converts to leuco-methylene blue, which is
colourless. Under the right conditions, cells and tissues are able to use
methylene blue in a way in which, in a sense, the dye substitutes for
oxygen. Instead of the respiratory processes resulting in the reduction of
oxygen to water, they cause the dye to convert to the leuco-form. The dye
gradually loses its colour, and by following the rate at which the blue fades,
it is possible to obtain a measure of the rate of respiration of the tissue in
the presence of the dye. When all the colour is gone, admission of oxygen
to the tube will result in the regeneration of the blue form of the dye, and
the experiment can be repeated. Requirements for various respiratory
substrates can be demonstrated, and much information about the effects
of substances which inhibit respiration can be gained. Results obtained by
the use of such simple equipment were later confirmed and extended.

When the problems associated with preparation of pure, active mito-chondrial fractions were solved, it offered a great encouragement to the development of the technical means for their study. Greatly improved techniques of spectroscopy, centrifugation and the introduction of the oxygen electrode led to an explosion of knowledge. The way in which

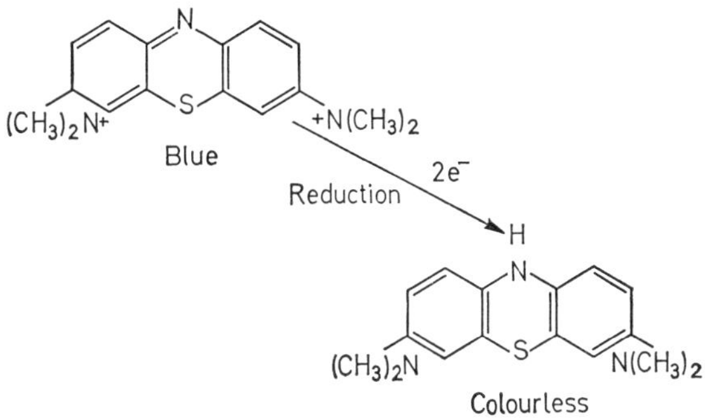

Fig. 2–4 The reduction of methylene blue to the colourless, leuco-form.

these instruments contributed to our understanding of the processes of respiration by mitochondria will be outlined in the remainder of this chapter and the next.

2.2 Oxidation and electron transfer

Historically, the term 'oxidation' was first used to describe those pro-cesses in which a substance combined with oxygen. Thus, the burning of carbon in air falls into this category quite readily:

$$C + O_2 \dashrightarrow CO_2$$

The term 'reduction' was similarly reserved for combination with hydrogen. As an example, under certain rigidly defined conditions, nitro-gen is reduced to ammonia:

$$N_2 + 3H_2 \dashrightarrow 2NH_3$$

However, the oxidation of hydrogen to yield water creates a number of semantic problems, as the reaction can be regarded either as an oxidation or a reduction, depending on which element is taken as the referent:

$$2H_2 + O_2 \dashrightarrow 2H_2O$$

Other definitions of oxidation were sought, and the best and most modern approach takes into account the transfer of electrons. Loss of electrons is oxidation; gain of electrons is reduction. Under this definition, the conversion of ferrous ion to ferric is oxidation:

$$Fe^{++} \dashrightarrow Fe^{+++} + e^-$$

ferrous   ferric + electron
ion   ion

The above equation underlies one of the most fundamental processes in respiration. Certain molecules associated with oxidation in cells contain iron. They are called cytochromes and their ability to undergo reversible oxidation-reduction reactions depends on the interconversion of ferrous and ferric ions attached to the molecules.

In cellular respiration, however, the problem assumes an even greater complexity because, in addition to ionic oxidation, the oxidation of organic molecules occurs. This is often achieved by dehydrogenation, the removal of hydrogen from the molecule, which is synonymous with oxidation. Dehydrogenation is mediated by specific catalysts or enzymes, and special electron acceptors. For example, succinic acid is oxidized to fumaric acid by an enzyme called succinic dehydrogenase:

$$
\begin{array}{ccc}
CH_2 \cdot COOH & & CH \cdot COOH \\
| & \dashrightarrow & \| \\
CH_2 \cdot COOH & & CH \cdot COOH
\end{array}
+ 2H^+ + 2e^-
$$

succinic acid   fumaric acid   protons electrons

The enzyme has two distinct parts; a protein portion and a flavin portion. The former is the catalyst, and the latter accepts electrons and protons from succinic acid.

Malic acid is converted to oxalaocetic acid:

$$
\begin{array}{ccc}
CH(OH) \cdot COOH & & CO \cdot COOH \\
| & + NAD^+ \dashrightarrow & | \\
CH_2 \cdot COOH & & CH_2 \cdot COOH
\end{array}
+ NADH + H^+
$$

malic acid   oxaloacetic acid

This reaction takes place in the presence of malic dehydrogenase. In this case, the acceptor of electrons and protons is not bound tightly to the enzyme, but it is still necessary for the reaction to occur. NAD^+ (nicotinamide adenine dinucleotide) is the oxidized form of the acceptor. In its reduced form, it is conventional to write it as $NADH + H^+$; it belongs to a group of substances which are ancillary to enzymes and are known as coenzymes or cofactors.

The electron flow may be more readily represented in the oxidation of hydroquinone:

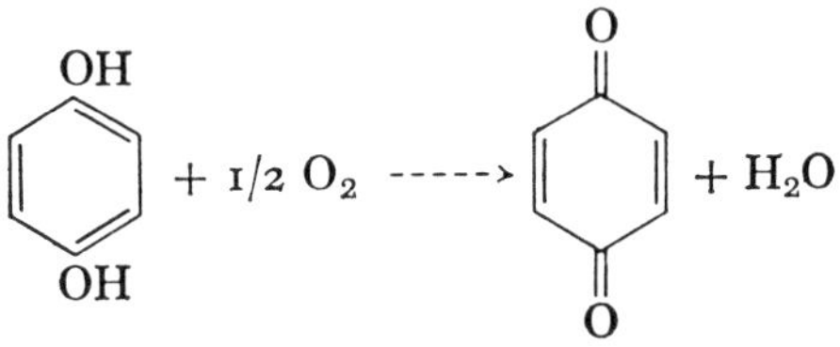

This reaction may be considered as a series of steps. The first is the dissociation of hydroquinone into its component ions:

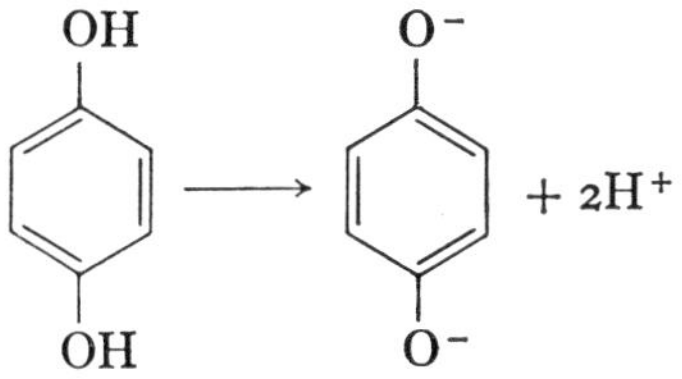

The second stage is the removal of electrons:

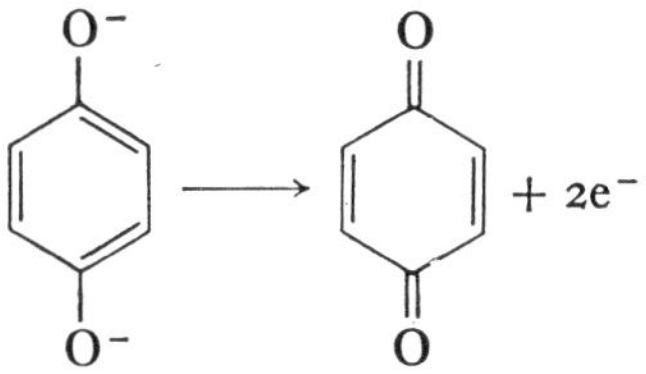

The electrons may then be accepted by another molecule. For example, if the ferric ion were the oxidant:

$$2e^- + 2Fe^{+++} \longrightarrow 2Fe^{++}$$

and the overall reaction becomes:

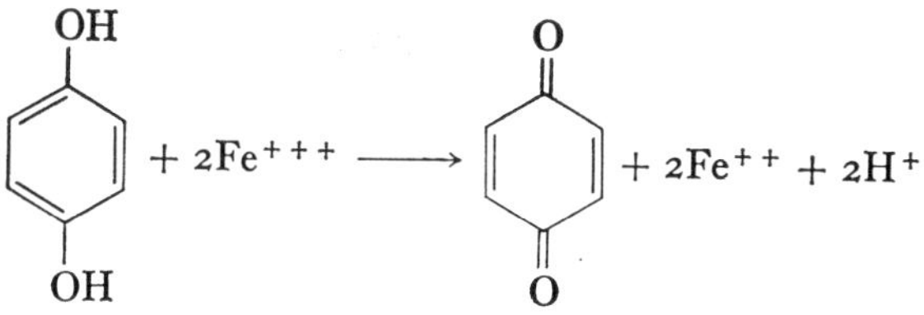

2

The hydroquinone reaction was deliberately chosen as an example because protons and electrons leave the parent molecule in well defined stages. In other cases, especially in biological systems, protons and electrons depart simultaneously as intact hydrogen atoms or as hydride ions, which are merely hydrogen atoms carrying an additional electron apiece.

2.3   The mitochondrion

Mitochondria occur in most cells, and are the major sites of respiratory activity within the cells. Understanding the structure of the mitochondrion provides a key to understanding its function. Before the advent of the electron microscope, mitochondria were considered to be structureless particles, perhaps vesicles, which were in some way implicated in oxidative processes. Their most spectacular property was their capacity to take up a vital dye, Janus Green B. The term 'vital' refers to its ability to stain only living tissue.

When the high resolution of the electron microscope became available, it was immediately found that the mitochondrion had an elaborate architecture. It was formed from an inner and an outer membrane. The surface of the inner membrane was much expanded, thrown into numerous folds or cristae, which served to increase the area. The cristae penetrated the whole of the interior of the mitochondrion. Between the cristae, and between the inner and outer membranes was a structureless material which was termed the matrix. Until recently, this was considered to be the extent of the structure. However, a new technique for the preparation of sections for examination by electron microscopy was applied to preparations of mitochondria.

The standard technique of staining for electron microscopy involves the deposition of heavy metals (which are electron-dense) on the membranes of the mitochondria themselves. Fernandez-Moran and Green introduced the method of negative staining. In this technique it is the space around the structures that is stained and not the structures themselves. The process leaves a 'negative' image of the specimen, and when mitochondria were subjected to this treatment, it was at once reported that numerous small knobs could be seen on the surface of the cristae. The knobs proved to be about the right size for the complexes of molecules of the enzymes which effect biological electron transport and phosphorylation.

The true nature of the knobs remains a subject for disagreement. Some workers have repeated the original work may times, but still others insist that they are artefacts due to the techniques employed, and that by a judicious selection of methods, knobs can be put on anything. The problem is still unresolved, but it has focused attention on the necessary configuration of enzymes within the mitochondrial structure.

Unlike many other enzyme systems, many of the enzymes associated with the mitochondrion are an integral part of its fabric. Loosely attached to the outer membrane are the enzymes of the tricarboxylic acid cycle. Attached to the inner membrane are the enzymes of electron transport and the electron carriers. It appears that in the matrix between the two membranes there is situated a mechanism which actively transports

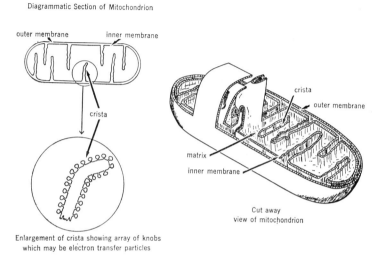

Diagrammatic Section of Mitochondrion

outer membrane   inner membrane

crista

crista

outer membrane

matrix

inner membrane

Cut away
view of mitochondrion

Enlargement of crista showing array of knobs
which may be electron transfer particles

Fig. 2–5 Diagram illustrating the structure of a mitochondrion.

electrons and protons backwards and forwards between the interior and exterior of the mitochondrion. The whole architecture of the mitochondrion is spatially organized to give a high degree of efficiency. Dehydrogenation reactions occur at its surface, and the electrons and protons pass to the interior; adenosine diphosphate (ADP) is also admitted. Electron transport then occurs via a highly integrated cytochrome system. The products, adenosine triphosphate (ATP) and water are returned to the outside.

It is the very property of high level organization which makes the mitochondrion such a difficult entity to study. Many enzymes, such as succinic dehydrogenase, and the electron transporting cytochromes, cannot be isolated without destroying the mitochondrion itself. This is the reason that many studies are concerned with the reassembling of the enzymes in order to determine the configuration that they enjoyed within the mitochondrion. It is one of the great difficulties faced by biochemists that many of its functions, including the most basic, that of oxidative phosphorylation, depend on maintaining the mitochondrion intact.

2.4   Electron transport in biological systems

It was early discovered that the pathway of glycolysis in animals and in yeast (in the latter organism, it is more usually referred to as fermentation; however, as the major differences are involved in the disposal of the end product, it is more convenient to use the single term) could not be detected in purified preparations of mitochondria. At the same time it was found that, with exceptions which will be considered in later chapters, the enzymes of the tricarboxylic acid cycle were generally present. A more detailed treatment of both metabolic pathways is given in an earlier volume in this series.*

The function of glycolysis and the tricarboxylic acid cycle is essentially one of maintenance. Together, they are the engines which keep the cell running, which ensure that there will be a sufficient quantity of chemical energy available for the cell's various activities. It is interesting to note that while the breakdown of glucose and polysaccharides is accomplished by a similar pathway in the majority of organisms, the tricarboxylic acid cycle has undergone modification in many cases. This lability of function may mean that the tricarboxylic acid cycle is less primitive than the glycolytic pathway. Another interpretation might be that not enough different organisms have yet been examined to permit the validity of the generalization!

Both pathways, whether separately or linked together, assist in the release of chemical energy which can be tapped by the organism. They comprise a metabolic grindstone, because they are concerned with the oxidation of larger molecules to smaller ones which can be further metabolized, or excreted as of no further use to the organism. Thus, under conditions of oxygen deficiency, oxidation of a molecule of glucose by glycolysis results in the production of two molecules of pyruvic acid and a net yield of two molecules of ATP. Under conditions of oxygen plenty, pyruvic acid is converted to acetyl co-enzyme A, and passed to the tricarboxylic acid cycle. The characteristic products of the activity of the tricarboxylic acid cycle are carbon dioxide (a large proportion of the carbon dioxide expired by terrestrial air-breathing animals is derived from this source), water, and by intercession of the electron transfer system, more than thirty molecules of ATP.

The process of oxidation is brought about by a series of dehydrogenation reactions which are included in the pathways. Thus, during glycolysis, glyceraldehyde-3-phosphate is converted to 1;3diphosphoglyceric acid; during tricarboxylic acid cycle activity iso-citric acid is converted to α-ketoglutaric acid, α-ketoglutaric acid is converted to succinic acid, and malic acid to oxaloacetic acid, all by reactions involving the phosphopyridine cofactors. Other pathways may also yield molecules of these

* Geoffrey R. Barker. Understanding the Chemistry of the Cell.

reduced cofactors. One dehydrogenation reaction in the tricarboxylic acid cycle, in which succinic is converted to fumaric acid, does not involve the participation of NAD; instead, the reaction is mediated directly by flavoprotein. It is essential that there be a mechanism for the reoxidation of the cofactors, in order that they may once again participate in cellular respiration.

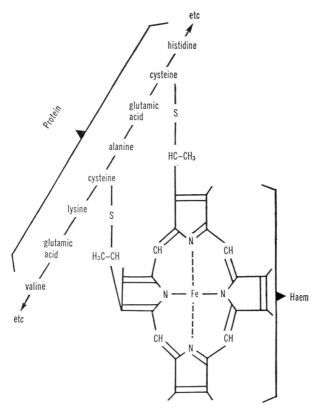

Fig. 2–6 Part of the structure of cytochrome c, a haemoprotein. The haem group comprises the four heterocyclic rings enclosing an iron atom. In the diagram the haem group should be envisaged as projecting at right angles to the plane of the paper. Cytochrome c has a molecular weight of about 12 000, and has only one haem group/molecule.

The first inklings of such a mechanism originated from the initial discoveries that dyes such as methylene blue were reduced by tissue preparations during respiration. There was no knowledge of the tricarboxylic acid cycle; several of the reactions had been discovered, but although Thunberg made an early, inspired attempt at the concept of biochemical cycles, it was an idea that did not gain much credence. Information about the cofactors involved was sketchy in the extreme. However, observations that the addition of the dye to media in which various preparations were being incubated caused a great acceleration of respiration made it clear that there must be some substance, analogous to the dye, which occurred naturally in cells, and which had a similar capacity for oxidation and reduction.

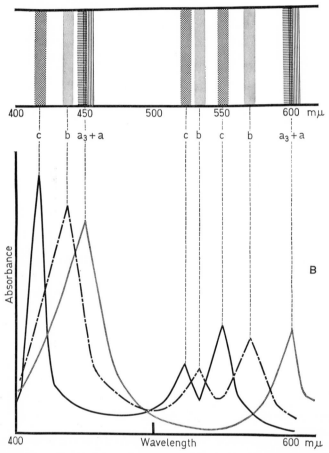

Fig. 2–7   The absorption of visible light by cytochromes. The upper diagram shows the distribution of dark bands in the visible spectrum when a suspension of oxygen deficient cells is viewed through a hand spectroscope. The lower diagram shows how each reduced cytochrome contributes to the pattern. Similar traces are obtained during spectrophotometry, as difference spectra.

There grew up two schools of thought. The first was that of Wieland, who maintained that the dehydrogenation step was of paramount importance; the second was that of Warburg, who thought that the reduction of oxygen was of greater significance. Warburg's insight led him to the postulation and identification of an iron containing respiratory enzyme which he called *Atmungsferment*, and the two schools remained at loggerheads until the rediscovery of the cytochromes by Keilin in 1923.

Cytochromes are complex proteins which contain iron incorporated into a haem group; hence they belong to a whole class of compounds, of which haemoglobin is also a member, called haemoproteins (Fig. 2–6). It was found that the cytochromes readily switched from the reduced condition to the oxidized one, given the right conditions, and vice versa. This was one way in which they proved similar to the dyes, and it became clear that the cytochromes were the bridge which would reconcile the apparently different philosophies of Warburg and Wieland. The two groups were merely studying different ends of the same process. An unexpected bonus was that the cytochromes were easily identifiable in the oxidized or the reduced conditions, because of their characteristic property of light absorption. Their absorption bands are quite distinct (Fig. 2–7).

In the first instance, only three cytochromes were recognized, and they were designated a, b and c. It has since been shown that there are, in fact, many more cytochromes, and the terms a, b and c now serve to designate the types into which they fall. In the mitochondrion, the cytochromes comprise a chain of molecules arranged and fixed in a specific sequence, which act as carriers of electrons and associated protons from the reduced cofactors to oxygen, with the formation of water. The cofactors thus become reoxidized and are available for further participation in oxidation reactions. The process can be illustrated as follows:

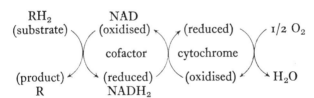

This is, of course, a general statement. In detail, it is a very complex system, parts of which are still not clearly understood.

The well-defined absorption bands which the cytochromes possess enabled Keilin to detect them with the hand spectroscope. The latter is a very simple device in which a prism is placed in front of a light source. The prism refracts the light so that when the source is viewed through it a spectrum can be seen. When a solution of cytochrome, c, for example, is interposed between the light source and the prism the viewer will still see the spectrum, but it will contain dark lines corresponding to those wavelengths of light which are absorbed by the cytochrome. In a suspension of yeast cells which has just been shaken, a composite picture of bands due to cytochromes, a, b and c in the oxidized form can be seen. If a reducing agent, such as sodium dithionite, is added to the suspension, oxygen is effectively removed from the solution. The observer then sees the bands due to the oxidized forms give way to those characteristic of the reduced forms of the cytochromes. The positions of the bands are shown in Fig. 2–7.

One of the great difficulties about making accurate measurements of the transmission of light through cell suspensions is that they are cloudy and much of the light is dispersed by the particles. In turbid solutions, the normal relationship between the amount of light absorbed by a solution and the concentration of the solute no longer holds. Although the mitochondrion is much smaller than a cell, it is still very much larger than even the largest of molecules, and so they also make turbid suspensions. Britton Chance and his colleagues therefore developed a spectrophotometer which used a very intense light source to transmit a beam through very dense suspensions, in order to measure small changes in the oxidative state of cytochromes in mitochondrial suspensions. Chance and his coworkers used difference spectra to a large extent. This was made possible because they incorporated a 'split beam' device into the instrument (Fig. 2–8). (A spectrophotometer differs in essence from the hand spectroscope in that, instead of an eye, there is at the end of the light path an extremely sensitive photomultiplier, which not only 'sees' the beam of light, but also enables the experimenter to measure its intensity very accurately.)

In order to understand how the system works, imagine a suspension of mitochondria in which it is necessary to determine the difference spectrum of the cytochromes. The preparation is split into two portions. One part is placed in a glass cell and bubbled with oxygen. In this cell, therefore, the cytochromes remain in the oxidized condition. The second portion is treated in exactly the same way, so that the contents of the two cells are, as nearly as possible, identical. One of them will act as a control or reference, the other as the test sample. They are both placed side by side in the spectrophotometer. Light emerges from the light source, and passes either through a prism or a diffraction grating to produce a spectrum. There is a screen containing a narrow slit placed in front of the prism or grating, and by rotating the latter, light of different wavelengths is allowed to pass through the slit. The slit is only wide enough to permit the passage of light of a single wavelength. The whole device is known as a monochromator and produces 'monochromatic' light. Monochromatic light now passes through a mirror device which splits the light beam into two. One beam passes through the reference suspension, the other through the test cell, and they then fall upon the surface of the photomultiplier. The photomultiplier measures the intensity of the light falling upon it from both cells and sends an impulse to a recorder which produces a trace, as each wavelength of

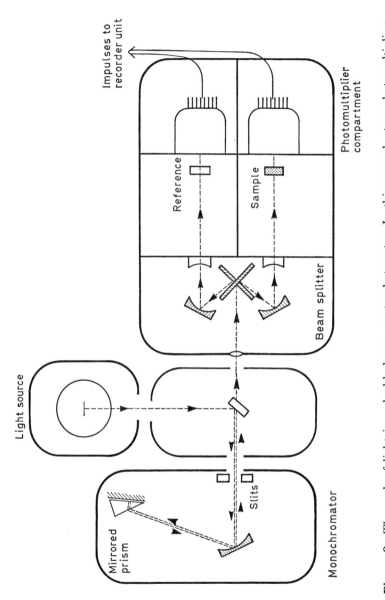

Fig. 2–8 The path of light in a double beam spectrophotometer. In this example, two photomultipliers are used; other systems employ only one.

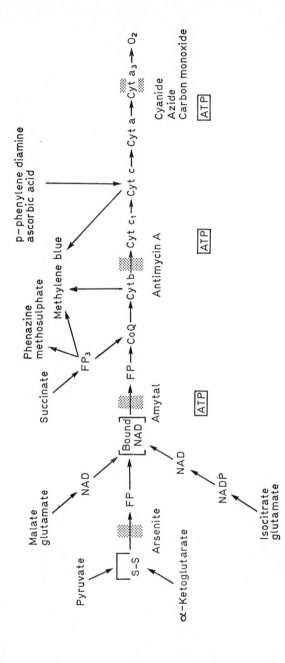

Fig. 2-9 Diagram of the electron transfer system, showing where common inhibitors act (shaded blocks) and where various compounds, natural or artificial, donate or accept electrons (indicated by the direction of the arrow).

light is automatically tested in turn. Because both suspensions are at the moment identical, the attenuation of each beam is also identical, and the trace will be a straight line along the zero level on the chart. If the suspension in the test cell is now reduced with sodium dithionite, there will be a difference between the reduced cytochromes in the test cell and the oxidized ones in the reference cell. The difference is transcribed on the chart for each wavelength. The resulting trace is a difference spectrum of oxidized versus reduced cytochromes, and appears as a series of peaks and troughs (Fig. 2–7). Any changes which occur in the test cell which are not related to the reduction process are automatically compensated for by similar changes occurring in the reference cell.

The use of techniques such as this, and the employment of specific inhibitors which interrupt the flow of electrons from one carrier to another has enabled the elucidation of the sequence of the main respiratory electron carriers in the chain. A simplified version of the respiratory chain is illustrated in Fig. 2–9.

Chance carried out a large number of elegant experiments to confirm this sequence. His group was able to determine, by direct methods, which carriers became reoxidized first as oxygen was admitted to a suspension in which the cytochromes were in a reduced condition. It involved recording the spectra at very short time intervals, and as the wave of oxidation swept along the chain, it was possible to see that cytochrome a was the first to become reoxidized, followed by c and so on, in reversed sequence.

In the respiratory chain illustrated in Fig. 2–9, the carriers of electrons are arranged in a sequence of increasing electropositiveness, with the dehydrogenase negative with respect to the cytochrome oxidase end. The electrons generated during dehydrogenation may therefore be considered to be flowing down a gradient, and it is during the passage of the negative electron to the positive end of the chain that something happens which is of the utomost importance to the cell. The energy associated with the change of potential is captured and used for the synthesis of the so-called high energy compound ATP, which is the fuel for the cell. This process of oxidative phosphorylation is described in the next chapter.

3.1 Introduction

It is a quite remarkable thing in the history of biochemistry that, although the concept of oxidative phosphorylation has a respectable antiquity—as long ago as 1906, the eminent chemists Harden and Young had shown that phosphate was an essential component in the conversion of glucose to alcohol by yeast—it still remains one of the most mysterious and contentious areas of study in 1969. It is even more surprising on comparison with the great advances which have been made in the field of molecular genetics, where a clear and fundamental concept emerged in the early 'fifties after a short but intensive period of study. *A priori*, it would seem that a complicated process like the transfer and retrieval of biological information based on the DNA molecule would not be easily unravelled. By the same token, the elucidation of a relatively simple chemical process like the synthesis of ATP from ADP ought certainly to reward diligent study. That it has not is, perhaps, due to the fact that there may be no simple unifying concept to explain oxidative phosphorylation, that the observed phenomenon is a composite of several different processes, and that the different ideas which are current in this area of biochemistry may each contribute a portion of the whole truth.

The term 'oxidative phosphorylation' is used almost exclusively to describe the reactions which lead to the synthesis of ATP. It implies that when, in a respiring system, a phosphate group is transferred to ADP an oxidation reaction is also involved. It is the mechanism by which energy from molecules of food is conveniently trapped and manipulated by all living organisms. ATP is the energy currency of cells and tissues, and may be used sparingly or wastefully, or stored or placed in the 'bank' by converting it to a phosphagen, which will yield ATP when it is required. It is only in the breakdown of a molecule of ATP that chemical energy becomes available to the cell for all its processes, whether chemical, mechanical or electrical. ATP is produced in constant supply by the mitochondria, and because of this, mitochondria are often found in large numbers in cells which expend energy in large quantities. An excellent example is insect flight muscle (Fig. 3–1), where the numerous mitochondria are very regularly arranged in close proximity to the muscle fibrils.

The general statement of the process of oxidative phosphorylation can be summarized as follows:

Eq. I. $\qquad AH_2 + B + ADP + P_i \rightleftharpoons A + BH_2 + ATP + H_2O$

where A and B are carriers of electrons, and AH_2 and BH_2 are the same carriers in the reduced condition. During the phosphorylation process which occurs during biological electron transfer, the roles of A and B are filled by the cytochromes. If the synthesis of ATP is to be achieved, there should be an electropotential difference between A and B sufficient to supply the energy required to yield one mole of ATP from one mole each of ADP and inorganic phosphate, P_i.

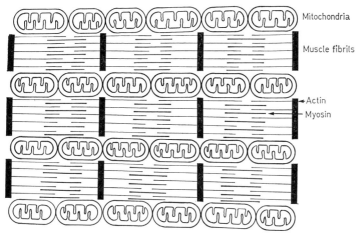

Mitochondria

Muscle fibrils

Actin

Myosin

Fig. 3-1   Diagram showing the intimate association and close array of mito-chondria and muscle fibrils in insect flight muscle.

Equation I may be expressed as the sum of two irreversible reactions, one of which is an oxidation, in which AH_2 is oxidized and B reduced:

Eq. II $$AH_2 + B \longrightarrow A + BH_2$$

and the other of which is the phosphorylation of ADP to yield ATP with the exclusion of a molecule of water:

Eq. III. $$ADP + P_i \longrightarrow ATP + H_2O$$

It is essential that the energy released in equation II is sufficient to drive the reaction indicated by equation III to the right; that is, in the direction of synthesis of ATP.

It must be clearly understood that these equations are only an abbreviated statement of an extremely complicated process. There are several theories which purport to give a chemical description of the reactions involved, and new data are continually being acquired. The remainder of this chapter will endeavour to summarize those concepts extant at the time of writing, although it is quite likely to be out of date at the time of publication because of the rapidity with which the field expands.

3.2   History

The history of modern biochemistry probably starts with the brothers

Büchner. In search of a tonic with medicinal properties, they came up
instead with a preparation of juices squeezed out of yeast cells which was
capable of carrying out fermentation. It was the first instance of a strictly
biological process occurring in the absence of living cells. Although this
observation was made at the end of the nineteenth century, it was not until
the first decade of the twentieth that some understanding of the chemistry
involved was gained. This understanding was largely due to the work of
Harden and Young who, using simple techniques such as heat deactivation
and dialysis, demonstrated that yeast juice was a mixture of many components. Among their most significant observations was the one mentioned earlier, that inorganic phosphate was required for fermentation to
take place in the cell free extract. Young subsequently separated a sugar
phosphate (fructose diphosphate) from the mixture; the identification of
glucose mono- and diphosphates soon followed.

During the period 1910 to 1930, the metabolic reactions of fermentation
were worked out in some detail. There were many more steps involved
than had earlier been appreciated, and it became apparent that the very
nature of fermentation permitted the release of the energy associated with
food or substrate molecules to take place in small packets. If all the energy
associated with the carbohydrate stored by a cell were released at once,
there would probably be sufficient heat generated to cook the cell contents;
thus, fermentation is a mechanism which allows the cell to dispose of small
amounts of energy at a time as it is released during the operation of the
metabolic pathway.

It was found that the energy required for the initial step in fermentation
(in effect, to prime the pathway) was derived from the oxidation of phos-
phoglyceraldehyde:

$$phosphoglyceraldehyde + pyruvate + H_2O$$
$$= phosphoglycerate + lactate$$

The energy conserved in this reaction was apparently stored as a phosphate
compound and later became available for the initial phosphorylation of
glucose.

Adenosine triphosphate was discovered by Lohmann in 1931, and it was
seen immediately that it could be implicated in the sort of reaction mentioned above. However, it was not until 1937 onwards that some inkling
was gained of the central position occupied by ATP. Kalckar was working
with cell-free homogenates of many mammalian tissues, and was able to
show that phosphorylation of glucose or adenosine monophosphate (AMP)
took place when homogenates were incubated with a variety of substrates
in air. He went on to show that if oxygen were excluded from the reaction
vessel, no such phosphorylation occurred. Lipmann later demonstrated
that a similar process took place when pyruvate was oxidized by bacteria,
and out of these experiments arose the term 'oxidative phosphorylation'.
From his studies, Lipmann evolved the concept of the high energy bond

which is often represented in formulae as a squiggle—for example ATP is sometimes written ADP∼P. The idea of high energy bonds applied principally to ATP, and was meant to indicate that when the terminal phosphate group is removed from the molecule, the energy associated with it was not merely dissipated, as in hydrolysis, but was transferred intact to some other molecule or system. Thus, ATP was envisaged as driving reactions which were endergonic; in other words, those reactions which required an input of energy to make them work were able to use ATP. Alternatively, the phosphate group with its associated energy could be transferred intact to another molecule for storage, which could then also be considered to possess a high energy bond.

It must be realized at this point that the concept of the high energy bond is a convenient fiction, and that the energy associated with the terminal phosphate bond of ATP is not very different from that associated with the remaining two bonds. The difference lies only in the fact that when the terminal phosphate group is transferred, the energy associated with maintenance of this bond in ATP is also transferred. The bond energy of the remaining phosphate groups in ATP is dissipated when the bond is broken. ATP is therefore a very useful molecule for injecting energy into a system.

Later, Ochoa and, separately, the Russian workers Belitzer and Tsibakova, made the most important observation that more than one atom of phosphorus was esterified—that is, more than one molecule of ATP was synthesized—for each atom of oxygen used by tissue preparations respiring aerobically. This led them to the conclusion that phosphorylation occurred not only at the level at which the substance being respired was oxidized (substrate level), but that it was also occurring at the level at which electrons derived from this oxidation were transported along the respiratory chain to oxygen. In order to measure the relative efficiencies of these systems, and to determine the exact quantitative relations of the process, the P/O ratio was invented. The P/O ratio may be defined as the number of molecules of ATP synthesized per atom of oxygen used. Thus, the oxidation of succinic acid to fumaric acid involves the formation of two molecules of ATP and the consumption of one atom of oxygen. The P/O ratio is therefore 2. In this example, oxidation takes place by the transport of electrons directly from succinic acid along the respiratory chain. In many oxidations, a cofactor, nicotinamide adenine dinucleotide (NAD) acts as an intermediary. The reoxidation of NAD is accomplished with a P/O ratio of 3.

The precise nature of the link between phosphorylation and the transport of electrons along the respiratory chain has exercised biochemists for the last thirty years. However, there is one sort of oxidative phosphorylation which does not directly involve the respiratory chain. It is called substrate linked phosphorylation, and about it there is a large measure of agreement.

3.3   Substrate linked phosphorylation

Substrate linked phosphorylation occurs at some point remote from the respiratory chain, and in close association with the substance that is oxidized, or substrate. In the known cases of substrate linked phosphorylation, the term AH_2 in equation I is fulfilled by an aldehyde, such as glyceraldehyde phosphate, or by either of the two keto acids, pyruvic or α-ketoglutaric. The latter reaction is particularly interesting as it involves guanosine diphosphate (GDP) as the initial acceptor of the high energy phosphate group, not ADP. The phosphate group is transferred to ADP to form ATP in a subsequent reaction.

The reaction involving glyceraldehyde phosphate is an integral part of the pathway of glycolysis, and is the first of two reactions in that pathway which result in the synthesis of ATP.

The overall reaction is:

$$R \cdot CHO + NAD^+ + ADP + P_i \rightleftharpoons R \cdot COOH + NADH + H^+ + ATP$$
$$\text{aldehyde} \qquad\qquad\qquad\qquad\qquad \text{acid}$$

There is an intermediate product, diphosphoglyceric acid, which is an acid anhydride of phosphoric and phosphoglyceric acids, and it may also be considered to be a high energy compound. It can be represented as $R \cdot COOP$. The overall equation can then be written as the sum of two separate reactions, which fit into the general statement for oxidative phosphorylation.

$$R \cdot CHO + NAD^+ + P_i \rightleftharpoons R \cdot COOP + NADH + H^+$$

$$R \cdot COOP + ADP \rightleftharpoons R \cdot COOH + ATP$$

Sum:

$$R \cdot CHO + NAD^+ + ADP + P_i \rightleftharpoons R \cdot COOH + \underbrace{NADH + H^+} + ATP$$

Eq. I $\qquad\qquad AH_2 + B + ADP + P_i \rightleftharpoons A + BH_2 + ATP$

The oxidation of pyruvate is also an integral part of the pathway of glycolysis. It is at this point that fermentation and glycolysis diverge, as pyruvic acid is converted to alcohol in the one and lactate in the other. In some microorganisms, the oxidation of pyruvate by NAD is coupled to phosphorylation thus:

$$CH_3 \cdot CO \cdot COOH + NAD^+ + ADP + P_i \rightleftharpoons$$
$$\text{pyruvic acid}$$
$$CH_3 \cdot COOH + NADH + H^+ + ATP + CO_2$$
$$\text{acetic acid}$$

The above reaction does not occur in animal tissues, where pyruvic acid is decarboxylated, and, in combination with coenzyme A, enters the tricarboxylic acid cycle as acetyl coenzyme A. Here, if oxygen is present, it undergoes further oxidation. Under anaerobic conditions, or when there is just not sufficient oxygen available, pyruvic acid is reduced to lactic acid, which accumulates.

The final case of substrate linked phosphorylation takes place within the tricarboxylic acid cycle itself. It is the reaction in which α-ketoglutaric acid is oxidized and decarboxylated (the process is called, imaginatively, oxidative decarboxylation) to give succinic acid. The overall equation is:

$$\underset{\text{α-ketoglutaric acid}}{HOOC \cdot CH_2 \cdot CH_2 \cdot CO \cdot COOH} + H_2O + NAD^+ + ADP \rightleftharpoons$$

$$\underset{\text{succinic acid}}{HOOC \cdot CH_2 \cdot CH_2 \cdot COOH} + CO_2 + NADH + H^+ + ATP + H_2O$$

and is the sum of several separate reactions which may be arranged to conform with the general scheme for oxidative phosphorylation described by equation I, except that guanosine triphosphate is the initial high energy product; ATP is synthesized in a subsequent reaction by a simple transfer of the phosphate group:

$$GTP + ADP \rightleftharpoons GDP + ATP$$

One final thing should be noted about the reactions described above. Only one molecule of ATP is derived from each of these substrate linked phosphorylations. In all cases, however, one of the products is reduced nicotinamide adenine dinucleotide, $NADH + H^+$. The latter can be reoxidized at the level of the respiratory chain, and one of the consequences of its reoxidation is the synthesis of three molecules of ATP.

3.4 Respiratory chain phosphorylation

Unlike the reactions described in the previous section, about which there is considerable unanimity, the process or processes involved in respiratory chain phosphorylation remain the subject of much polemical discussion. There are two broad categories into which the theories may be made to fit. The first category ascribes phosphorylation to strictly chemical processes, and prior to 1961, all efforts to explain it fell within its confines. In 1961, Mitchell proposed a revolutionary new hypothesis which was based on the fact that concentration gradients of hydrogen and hydroxyl ions could be established across the mitochondrial membrane, which is, of course, the location of the respiratory chain. Mitchell's hypothesis has become known as the 'Chemiosmotic Coupling Hypothesis' and was erected largely on physical principles rather than chemical ones. It is still being evaluated, but there is no doubt that, even if it is proved incorrect, it has resulted in a reappraisal of the more orthodox ideas and has stimulated the gathering of fresh data in an effort to test it.

The sequence of reactions in the respiratory chain, as far as they are known, has been described in the previous chapter. Along the chain's length, there are three sites at which phosphorylation is known to occur, and during the passage of electrons past these points, three molecules of ATP are synthesized from three molecules of inorganic phosphate and three molecules of ADP.

The first site at which ATP is generated is at the point where the reoxidation of NADH takes place. The second is situated between cytochromes b and c_1, and the third is associated with cytochromes a and a_3. The chemical hypotheses suggest that at these points a complex of enzymes is located whose overall effect is to accomplish the phosphorylation described by equation I.

Many different techniques have been tried in an effort to elucidate the exact stages by which phosphorylation takes place. One of the major tools of the biochemist is the use of inhibitors, poisons which have, it is hoped, a specific effect on the system under examination. This ideal is rarely realized. The rationale for these experiments is that if the nature of the inhibition can be determined, then some insight into the normal reaction mechanism may be gained. Although it is a philosophy reminiscent of destructive monkey curiosity, an enormously large amount of information about reactions has repaid mathematical analysis of their variations in the presence of numerous inhibitors. Studies of the nature of inhibition form a major part of the science of enzyme kinetics.

In the case of the respiratory chain phosphorylations, much information has been gathered by the use of a class of inhibitors known as uncoupling agents. Many substances fall in this category; notable among them are the thyroid hormone, aspirin derivatives and barbiturates. However, the effect that they produce is not as marked as that produced by a substance, called 2,4-dinitrophenol, which is used routinely in experiments on oxidative phosphorylation.

An uncoupling agent, as its name suggests, is an inhibitor which exerts its effect by disassociating (uncoupling) the respiratory and phosphorylative functions of the electron transport system. It can best be illustrated by an analogy. Imagine an elongated drive belt meshing at three points along its length with three smaller drive wheels. The latter are, in turn, linking to other devices so that the driving power is transmitted from the belt, through the drive wheels to other machines. The other machines may be actually doing work, or they may be used to store energy, by recharging batteries, for example. The drive belt can thus be compared with the respiratory chain, and the mechanisms coupled to it represent the complex of phosphorylating enzymes. The uncoupling agent can then be considered to be a sort of clutch mechanism which can put the drive out of gear (Fig. 3–2). It might also be imagined that when the hypothetical drive is freed from the restraint imposed upon it by the energy handling devices, it will accelerate. This is exactly what happens when the respiratory chain is freed from the restraint imposed upon it by the phosphorylation mechanism; it races. Transfer of electrons along it, as measured by the uptake of oxygen, is increased under the influence of uncoupling agents.

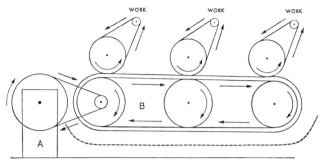

Fig. 3-2 A fanciful representation of oxidative phosphorylation. The motor, A, is driving a continuous belt B, which, in turn, is driving three smaller engines. The output of the latter is used either for doing mechanical work, or for storing energy, perhaps in recharging batteries. As in all analogies, the correspondence is by no means exact. However, the motor A can be compared with the processes by which foodstuffs are broken down to molecules small enough to enter the respiratory chain, the drive belt can be compared with the chain itself, and the smaller engines with phosphorylation reactions. If the drive belt were to be lowered to the level of the dotted line it would uncouple from the small engines. This could be achieved, either by suitable controls during normal working, or by throwing a spanner in the works 2, 4-dinitrophenol is a spanner.

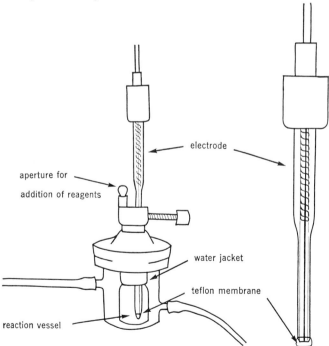

Fig. 3-3 Diagram of an oxygen electrode apparatus.

Uncoupling occurs 'naturally', as well as in the presence of toxic agents like dinitrophenol. One of the criteria of a good preparation of mitochondria is that in the absence of uncoupling agents it shall have a low oxygen uptake—that is, it is 'tightly coupled'. The degree of coupling may be determined experimentally by the use of an oxygen electrode attached to a recorder, which is illustrated, together with a specimen record, in Figs. 3–3 and 3–4. The electrode measures the rate at which oxygen is taken up from solution by a suspension of mitochondria in a closed, air-tight vessel. When an uncoupling agent is added, the uptake of oxygen and hence the slope of the trace increases. The same apparatus can be used for showing that the respiration rate also depends to a large extent on the presence of a sufficient quantity of acceptor for high energy phosphate groups, ADP. In the absence of ADP, mitochondria respire at a steady rate which is increased by the addition of the acceptor. This affords a ready method for the determination of P/O ratios, as the experimenter

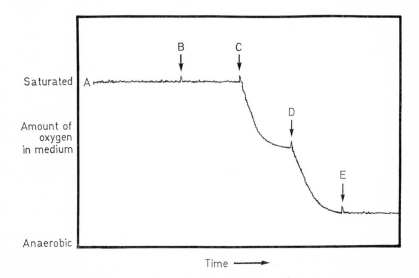

Fig. 3–4 A typical oxygen consumption trace obtained with an oxygen electrode attached to a recorder. Mitochondria in the resting state have little or no oxygen consumption (A). Substrate is added at point B. If the preparation is a good one, there should be no effect on the oxygen uptake. At point C, a known quantity of ADP is introduced into the vessel. The trace is immediately deflected downwards, showing that oxygen is being taken up. When all the ADP has been utilized, the trace stabilizes at a new level. Further addition of ADP (D) results in an identical response. A third addition of ADP (E) elicits no response as all the substrate has now been consumed. The time taken is about five minutes, and from these results a P/O ratio may be calculated.

knows how much ADP he has added and can compute the amount of oxygen used from the trace on his chart.

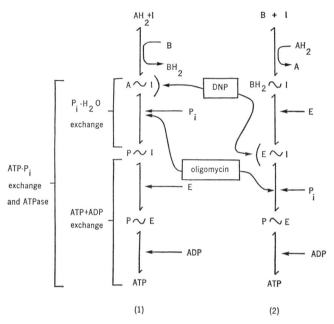

(1)   (2)

Fig. 3–5   Two theories of oxidative phosphorylation based on hypothetical intermediates, whose existence is deduced from experiments with inhibitors and the exchange reactions. The first scheme is due to Wadkins and Lehninger, the second to Chance and Williams. Both depend on the formation of high energy intermediates (A ∼ I, P ∼ I, P ∼ E; BH₂ ∼ I, E ∼ I, and P ∼ E) for which there is no direct evidence.

E represents enzyme molecule, and I represents an unknown chemical substance (occasionally designated C or X). DNP (dinitrophenol) is thought to cause the breakdown of A ∼ I to A + I (or E ∼ I to E + I). Oligomycin, which is not an uncoupler, is thought to inhibit the reaction in which inorganic phosphate becomes incorporated into an organic intermediate with a high energy phosphate bond.

The partial reactions are also illustrated in this scheme and are thought to derive from the activity of parts of the reaction sequence as indicated (From LEHNINGER, A. L., 1964, *The Mitochondrion*, Benjamin, New York and Amsterdam).

Studies of the effects of uncouplers, of inhibitors of electron transport such as antimycin, and of inhibitors of phosphorylation have led to the establishment of theories of oxidative phosphorylation based on the formation of hypothetical high energy intermediates. In order to explain some of the data, a multistep phosphorylation sequence has been postulated. It is to a large extent supported by studies of the so-called partial reactions, using components containing radioactive atoms as 'markers'. The partial reactions are thought to represent steps in the overall ATP synthesis, and include observations on the exchange between inorganic phosphate and the terminal phosphate in ATP, and the exchange of oxygen between inorganic phosphate and water. Another important characteristic of mitochondria is their ability, when they have been allowed to stand for some time, to break down ATP to ADP and inorganic phosphate. This is called ATPase activity and it is thought that it may be the phosphorylating reaction acting in the reverse direction.

Attempts to extract the enzymes responsible for phosphorylation from mitochondria, and to isolate the hypothetical intermediates have so far not been crowned with success. When an enzyme preparation is found to be capable of phosphorylation, it usually transpires that it is a very complex preparation indeed, and contains mitochondrial membrane and a number of the other ancillary mitochondrial enzymes. No pure or soluble preparation has been achieved. A major problem is that mitochondria readily lose their ability to carry out phosphorylation reactions while retaining their ability to transport electrons. Thus, the success of any technique for the isolation of the phosphorylating enzymes is jeopardized by the very act of preparation. It is a prime example of the 'observer effect', where the act of observation modifies the events observed. As twenty years of research of the most intensive kind have not lent too much substance to the chemical theories, which are based solely on circumstantial evidence, it may be that attention had better be given to different conceptions of the phenomena of oxidative phosphorylation.

The chemi-osmotic coupling hypothesis may provide just such an alternative. It is a revolutionary, but, in its general outlines, a simple idea which does away with the need for ephemeral and occult chemical intermediates. In brief, Mitchell suggests that phosphorylation is a function of the mitochondrial membrane and that efforts to study the process in the absence of the membrane are therefore meaningless. The hypothesis is best illustrated by diagram (Fig. 3–6). It suggests that the enzymes responsible for oxidative phosphorylation consist only of those known to occur in the respiratory chain together with the electron carriers, and an enzyme which synthesizes ATP from ADP and inorganic phosphate. Because the latter is so often manifested in the reverse role, it is called ATPase. In order for phosphorylation to occur, the enzymes must be situated in their correct places in an undamaged mitochondrial membrane. The first enzyme and the last enzyme in the respiratory chain, namely, the dehydrogenase and cytochrome oxidase, must also be asymmetrically arranged in the membrane.

Thus, the net effect of the passage of two electrons along the respiratory chain during the oxidation of a molecule of substrate is the build-up of two hydrogen ions on the outside of the membrane and two hydroxyl ions on the inside. The repetition of this process results in the formation of an ion or pH gradient across the membrane. The ATPase is so arranged that, during the formation of ATP from ADP and inorganic phosphate, the hydroxyl are passed to the *outside* and the hydrogen ions to the *inside* of the membrane. Thus the effect of the activity of the ATPase is to abolish the ion gradient across the membrane resulting from the activity of the respiratory chain. By establishing the ion gradient, respiratory chain activity 'forces' the ATPase to act in the direction of ATP synthesis.

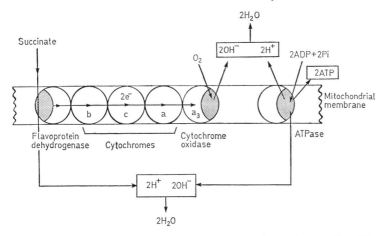

Fig. 3–6 Principle of Mitchell's hypothesis of chemiosmotic coupling. The dehydrogenation of succinate causes the delivery of protons to the lower side of the membrane, whereas the reduction of oxygen causes delivery of the hydroxyl ions to the upper side of the membrane, because of the asymmetric orientation of the active sites of succinic dehydrogenase and cytochrome oxidase, respectively. The accumulation of these ions at opposite sides of the membrane then 'pulls' the reverse action of ATPase, by causing the asymmetric extraction of protons and hydroxyl ions from ADP and P_i in the opposite directions. Since the ion product $[H^+][OH^-]$ is very low (1×10^{-14}), the formation of ATP from ADP and P_i may be driven by electron transport, providing that the mitochondrial membrane is impermeable to H^+ and OH^-. Redrawn from Lehninger (loc. cit.).

There are, of course, flaws in the attractive simplicity of the hypothesis; there are many observations reported in the literature which it does not satisfactorily explain. Among these is the ability of certain mitochondrial fragments to carry out oxidative phosphorylation. Perhaps the greatest contribution that the chemi-osmotic coupling hypothesis has made to the study has been in its nuisance effect. Many workers are now devoting their attention to the devising of the critical experiments to confirm the hypothesis. At the time of writing no new data to resolve the conflict have been uncovered, although an enormous amount of information has been gained.

Doing Without Oxygen

4.1 Aerobiosis and anaerobiosis

Current theories of the origin of life suggest that it occurred under conditions of reducing atmosphere—an atmosphere, that is, containing high proportions of hydrocarbons and no oxygen. There was, therefore, no alternative to the evolution of anaerobic metabolic pathways, and it is probable that the earliest biochemical systems transferred energy by substrate linked processes. At a later date—and it seems obvious that this part of the origin of life must have occupied a time span greater than that subsequently required for the whole of organic evolution since the Cambrian—the adoption of the phosphate group as an energy carrier must have occurred, with the evolution of storage molecules such as ATP.

The pathway of glycolysis is an excellent example of a highly organized enzyme system which embodies the principles set down in the preceding paragraph. The end product of glycolysis under anaerobic conditions is lactic acid, derived from pyruvic acid; the similar pathway of alcoholic fermentation results in the production of alcohol from acetaldehyde. These differences apart, the two pathways have a generic similarity, and even the reasons for the production of the acid and the alcohol are identical. Each reaction enables the reoxidation of cofactors which have become reduced in preceding reactions. Pyruvic acid and acetaldehyde are therefore acting as electron acceptors.

The ultimate fates of the acid and the alcohol are of considerable importance. In the case of fermenting yeast, alcohol accumulates in the medium until it reaches a concentration sufficient to inhibit any further fermentative activity on the part of the fungus. On the other hand, although lactic acid may accumulate in animals respiring anaerobically, it may subsequently be used; for example, it could be reconverted to carbohydrate, or, if the animal switches back to aerobic respiration, it could be oxidized further. It may also be excreted.

When, in the course of the evolution of life on Earth, free oxygen became available in large quantities, it seems that a further function was added to the anaerobic ones. Instead of using the end product of the anaerobic pathway as the ultimate electron acceptor, a whole new series of reactions evolved which culminated in the transfer of electrons to oxygen, and thus the mechanism for the reoxidation of reduced coenzymes and for the generation of ATP came to depend on the presence of molecular oxygen. This, no doubt, was influenced initially by the catalytic effect of iron on oxidative processes, and further evolution resulted in the incorporation of the iron into even more effective catalytic molecules. The cytochromes and flavoproteins appeared, and presumably at a later stage still, became incorporated into fixed structures which were the forerunners of the mitochondrion.

Implicit in this description is the commonly accepted conception of the difference between anaerobic and aerobic metabolism. In anaerobic metabolism, the synthesis of ATP occurs only at the substrate level, whereas aerobic metabolism is mediated by a system of iron-containing catalysts which transfer electrons to oxygen, and ATP synthesis occurs at substrate level *and* at the level of the electron transport system. Thus, instead of accumulating lactic acid, oxygen users can oxidize pyruvic acid directly.

But there is nothing magic about oxygen. Its great advantages are that there is a lot of it, that it is rather a small molecule, that it gets inside the organism readily and that it has the right redox potential. The last is most important, because any molecule which is transportable to the site of the terminal reaction of the electron transport system, and which has the correct redox potential, may substitute for oxygen. Use is made of this fact in experiments to determine the sequence of components of the electron transport system in isolated preparations of mitochondria. Various dyes and other molecules, such as methylene blue, phenazine methosulphate and various of the tetrazolium blue compounds, have redox potentials comparable with those of components of the electron transport system, and are able to accept electrons from it. Other substances, such as ascorbic acid and *p*-phenylene diamine, also with similar redox potentials, are able to donate electrons to the chain. As they operate in the electron transfer system at different points, by virtue of their differing redox potentials, judicious use of these substances in mitochondrial preparations, followed by spectrophotometric examination of the reaction mixture, can determine which components of the cytochrome system are by-passed by these molecules. From this it is possible to build up a picture of the components of the system.

These experiments demonstrate quite clearly that it is not unreasonable to envisage naturally occurring pathways of respiration which involve cytochromes, but in which the ultimate electron acceptors are molecules other than oxygen. They would be anaerobic pathways in the accepted sense, as the organisms possessing them would be independent of oxygen. End products would be formed, from which (if they were capable of being oxidized further, even though released into the environment) an obvious parallel could be drawn with glycolysis. The pathway would not, however, differ fundamentally from the principle of the orthodox cytochrome system.

It is necessary to point out one other pitfall. Anaerobiosis implies that oxygen does not participate in the molecular events of respiration, but it does not necessarily mean that anaerobic organisms have absolutely no requirement for oxygen. Some parasites, for example, need oxygen for growth to take place. Many other non-respiratory processes require oxygen;

oxidation of amino acids, tanning of many insect cuticles and collagen synthesis are three examples.

The remainder of this chapter will be devoted to consideration of those animals which, while they are true aerobes, are adapted to survival for relatively short periods during which they have reduced or no access to molecular oxygen. Anaerobiosis may be imposed on the animal in one of two ways; either the environment denies oxygen to it, or the limitation is imposed by a change in its own metabolism. The evolution of the ability to survive such deprivation has progressed both in the direction of the conservation and efficient distribution of residual supplies of oxygen in the body of the organism—modifications which tend not to be modifications of metabolic pathways, but rather to use existing systems in somewhat different ways combined with physiological innovation—and in the direction of biochemical innovation, where adaptation at the level of the metabolic pathway appears to take place.

4.2   The oxygen debt

The metabolic systems which have been described in Chapters 2 and 3 are essentially similar in all organisms which inhabit environments in which there is an abundance of oxygen. It is true that only relatively few animals have been studied, and conclusions are based largely on mammalian and bacterial studies, but the additional evidence from the majority of other vertebrates does not seriously call these findings into question. In invertebrate animals, the generalization may not be quite so valid, but invertebrate material is not easy to handle, and there is often not enough of it, and work lags far behind that mentioned above. There is some evidence which suggests that differences may occur in invertebrates occupying environments low in oxygen, but in obligate oxygen users, mechanisms may not differ too widely from those found in the mammals. Examples of those animals which suffer oxygen deprivation as a way of life, imposed from without by the external environment, are examined in Chapter 5.

One of the more important problems that all oxygen users have to face from time to time is, how to sustain life if temporarily deprived of oxygen. An active mammal dies in very few minutes if it is denied oxygen. A hibernating mammal, cold blooded reptile, amphibian or fish may, under certain circumstances, survive for several hours in the absence of oxygen; but the eventual outcome is the same. It is clear, therefore, that any mechanism which permits the organism to survive short periods of anoxia unharmed will have great survival value. As an example, the newborn human infant survives unharmed for considerably longer periods of oxygen deprivation than an adult under the same conditions—but only in the minutes immediately preceding and following its birth. In the case of slow deliveries, this character obviously contributes greatly to survival.

In animals which inhabit environments of low or fluctuating oxygen

ension, it is a condition of life that they should be capable of the main-
enance of normal body activities during prolonged periods of anoxia
which are the normal conditions of their environment. Organisms which
are adapted to life in atmospheres or baths containing high concentrations
of oxygen, and where oxygen deprivation is relatively rare, do not experience
he same pressures. Tolerance of low oxygen tensions may need to extend
or, perhaps, several minutes at the most.

If an animal is deprived of oxygen, its electron transport system, if it
conforms to the classic pattern, becomes useless. ATP is no longer
synthesized, and the oxidation processes normally carried on by the tricarboxylic acid cycle can no longer occur. This, in turn, means that the
erminal products formed through the activity of glycolysis, which is
ndependent of oxygen, will accumulate. Unless the organism possesses
some mechanism for disposing of the most important of these products,
pyruvic acid and the reduced phosphopyridine nucleotides, intermediary
metabolism will come to a halt. The first problem, therefore, is to maintain
he supply of ATP for sustaining the activities of the animal, and the second
problem is how to compensate for the sudden drop in the concentrations
of the oxidized cofactors.

Although total deprivation of oxygen is an infrequent occurrence for
aerobic organisms, the occasions on which certain of their tissues are called
upon to act aerobically are not rare. A good example is a human sprinter.
His circulatory system cannot possibly supply the total oxygen requirements of his leg muscles, so the muscles switch from the aerobic mode to
the anaerobic mode of respiration. In the process, they deplete any stores
of oxygen which reside in the muscle myoglobin, and any stores of ATP
and creatine phosphate. For its ATP the muscle depends largely on the
activity of the glycolytic pathway. Under normal circumstances, this would
result in the accumulation of large quantities of pyruvic acid.

Pyruvic acid is prevented from accumulating by its conversion to lactic
acid. In a single reaction, the end product of the metabolic pathway is
removed so that there is no longer any danger of it inhibiting the process
which brought about its formation (product inhibition), and reduced
pyridine nucleotides are reoxidized:

$$CH_3 \cdot CO \cdot COOH + NADH + H^+ \rightleftharpoons CH_3 \cdot CH(OH) \cdot COOH + NAD^+$$

pyruvic acid   lactic acid

Under physiological conditions, the equilibrium is heavily in favour of
the formation of lactic acid. Tissues tolerate relatively high concentrations
of it.

Thus, when the human sprinter (or any other mammal, for that matter)
is in action, an insufficient quantity of oxygen arrives at the muscles; the
muscles exhaust what stores they have and turn to lactic acid production.
In doing so, they accumulate an 'oxygen debt' because the amount of
lactic acid produced is equivalent to an amount of oxygen in excess of that

available. This debt is normally discharged in the minutes subsequent to the activity. Panting is a way of getting more oxygen into the sprinter to pay off the debt incurred by his muscles. When all the lactic acid has been oxidized, the debt is repaid.

There are, however, more ways than one of surmounting the enforced periods of anaerobiosis. Many animals repay the oxygen debt after deprivation; pond snails, marine bivalves, some insects, planarians and annelids and many of the more active vertebrates fall into this category. Some organisms, on the other hand, excrete the lactic acid and so avoid paying the oxygen debt altogether. These are the animals which are commonly thought of as anaerobic, such as the worms parasitic in the intestines of mammalian hosts. Usually, however, such parasites are not restricted to the single acid but, in addition, excrete a variety of others, such as the methyl butyric and the valeric acids. The mechanisms which are employed to avoid the necessity of repaying the debt are considered in the next chapter.

Still other organisms repay only part of the debt, and in these some of the lactate which has accumulated in their muscles is reconverted to carbohydrate for storage.

It is clear that the biochemical key to the problem of the switch from aerobic to anaerobic metabolism must lie with the enzyme responsible for the interconversion of pyruvic and lactic acids. The nature of the enzyme responsible, lactic dehydrogenase, is still not clearly understood, but it is becoming more apparent that one of its roles is to assist in metabolic regulation. Recent research has shown that a single molecule of the enzyme is composed of four polypeptide chains. A polypeptide chain is a chain of amino acids linked together in the same way as they are in a protein, but in insufficient numbers to give a molecular weight consistent with that of a molecule of a protein. The molecule is also not big enough to possess a number of the other peculiar characteristics of proteins. However, two or more such polypeptide chains can become attached to produce a proper protein. The polypeptide chains of lactic dehydrogenase have been designated either H or M.

When a supposedly homogeneous preparation of lactic dehydrogenase is extracted from a tissue such as muscle, it will catalyse the reaction in which pyruvic and lactic acids are interconverted as if it were indeed a single enzyme. If, however, the preparation is dissolved in a suitable buffer and absorbed onto a plate of gel prepared in the same buffer, and if an electric current is permitted to pass through the treated plate, something unexpected happens. Instead of the enzyme traversing the plate as a single substance, by virtue of the charge it carries, it may separate into as many as five components. This means that the hitherto homogeneous preparation is, in fact, heterogeneous and the components differ with respect to the charges they carry. If the five components are now eluted from the plate of gel, it will be found that they are all capable of carrying out the lactic dehydrogenase reaction. They are therefore termed 'iso-enzymes'.

The isoenzymes all consist of the four polypeptide chains mentioned earlier, but they differ with respect to the proportions of the H and M chains that they contain. Thus, the five isoenzymes of lactic acid corre-spond to the five possible combinations of the H and M polypeptides which

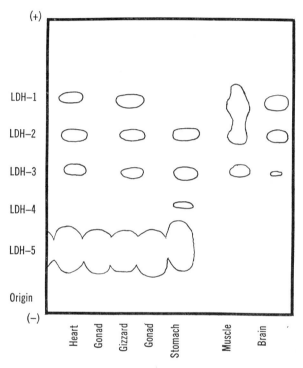

Fig. 4–1 Diagram to show the distribution of isoenzymes of lactic de-hydrogenase in tissues from the horseshoe crab (from E. J. MASSARO, *Science*, **167**, 994, 1970).

form the enzyme. The five possibilities range from the all-H form, H—H—H—H, through the intermediate forms, H—H—H—M, H—H—M—M, H—M—M—M, to the all-M form, M—M—M—M, and the various combinations of charges result in their different mobilities during electrophoretic separation. This does not necessarily exclude the pos-sibility that there may be other isoenzymes of lactic acid which bear the same charge and hence are not separated.

The significance of the observation that the different isoenzymes have different combinations of the H and M polypeptide chains resides in their behaviour during the reaction. Lactic dehydrogenases which have a high proportion of isoenzymes which contain a predominant number of the H-polypeptide chains are more sensitive to substrate inhibition than those lactic dehydrogenases which are composed of isoenzymes in which M polypeptide chains predominate. In practical terms, this means that i pyruvic acid is added to a test tube which contains already a reaction mixture consisting of the H-containing enzymes and pyruvic acid, and o course the product, lactic acid, then the result will be a slowing up of the rate at which pyruvic is converted to lactic acid. Conversely, the M-containing enzymes continue to function in relatively high concentrations o pyruvic acid.

If the *in vitro* findings can be applied to *in vivo* conditions, a transference which is always fraught with pitfalls, it would seem that the H enzymes would be inhibited under conditions which would result in a build-up o pyruvic acid. These conditions obtain in the absence of oxygen, when pyruvic acid can no longer be oxidized via the tricarboxylic acid cycle Thus, tissues which are capable of anaerobic respiration might be expected to contain enzymes which are mainly M.

The hypothesis is supported by the facts. Cardiac muscle is exclusively aerobic, and H forms predominate in its lactic dehydrogenase. In skeletal muscle, which is frequently called upon to act anaerobically, there are relatively greater amounts of the M enzymes. It therefore appears that the pattern of lactic dehydrogenase inhibition represents an important control point in the regulation of anerobic and aerobic metabolism.

4.3   Diving animals

Diving mammals provide some excellent examples of how all levels o organization can contribute to the solution of problems posed by environ ment. In the preceding section, survival for very short periods of oxyger deprivation has been discussed. Here, the mechanisms which enable whales to sound for periods of more than an hour, and for seals and beaver to remain submerged for twenty minutes without harm, while the best tha man can manage is two or three minutes, will be briefly considered. In thi context it is also interesting to note that the physiological compensatory patterns established by highly trained human divers are similar to those normally present in diving mammals.

There is one great distinction between divers and non-divers. When submerged, the diver is relaxed and seemingly comfortable; the non-diver struggles wildly. Quite apart from the aspect of familiarity with the situa tion, it is an example of one of the levels of adaptation possessed by the diver; behavioural characteristics (including economy of effort) which permit prolonged submersion. The key to successful diving among the mammals appears to lie in physiological rather than biochemical adapta tion, and includes modified behaviour, modified circulation and modified gas exchange. Parallel mechanisms appear in animals of the other verte-brate classes.

Diving mammals do not use oxygen at lower rates than terrestrial mammals; it is the distribution of oxygen which is important, and the efficiency with which it is used. The amount of air replaced in the lungs with each breath may be as high as 80 per cent in diving mammals; this is four times the proportion of exchange accomplished by man. In most other characteristics, however, man compares quite favourably. A notable departure is that muscles of divers often contain very much more myoglobin per unit weight. Myoglobin is a haemoprotein closely related to haemoglobin, and like the later, combines with oxygen in such a way that it is readily released when the oxygen tensions in the tissues drop below a critical level. In whales, myoglobin may account for some 40 per cent of the total oxygen stored in the animal's body. It cannot, however, supply the oxygen that would be required in a prolonged dive, as it is all used during the first ten minutes of submersion. Instead, the muscles of the whale turn to anaerobic activity.

The most economical way in which stored oxygen can be used is by routing it to the tissues which are most sensitive to anoxia. The brain, nervous system and heart are much more susceptible than other tissues, and in order to keep them supplied with oxygen, a most remarkable circulatory mechanism has evolved. Nearly thirty years ago, Scholander demonstrated that, in seals, the circulation of the blood to the muscles was interrupted during diving; at the same time, the rate of heart beat was slowed. Lactic acid was retained in the muscles during the dive; when the dive was completed, at the first breath, the heart speeded up again and lactic acid flooded the circulatory system showing that circulation to the muscles had been restored. The shutting off of the blood supply to the muscles, by constriction of the blood vessels, conserves oxygen which is transported by the reduced circulation to the brain and heart, which have the greater need. It is interesting to note that a similar phenomenon occurs in man. Constriction of the blood vessels in the muscles accompanied by a reduced rate of heart beat occurs in professional shell divers.

Similar modifications are seen in the circulatory systems of a variety of diving birds, including cormorants, puffins and auks, and in alligators and snakes. In fish, the same changes have been observed when the flying fish 'dives' from its normal watery environment into the air. On the other hand, the Australian mud skipper is a fish that spends most of its time on land. When it enters the water, it reacts in the same way. A final example may be drawn from man. When the human infant 'dives' from its comfortable, intra-uterine, fluid-filled world into the world of the air breathers, it experiences the same physiological reactions. They extend, by a few minutes, the safe period that a new born infant has in which to start breathing. The baby can withstand this critical period without injury in the vast majority of cases. A contributory factor is that the brain of a new-born baby is far less susceptible to periods of anoxia than that of an adult.

4.4   Intermediate cases

One of the problems of any scientific study is that nothing is ever wholly black or wholly white. The distinction between short term and long term survival or oxygen deprivation is, at best, a fuzzy one. Short term solutions provide an answer to anoxia for periods of up to a maximum of two hours or so. The long term solutions equip the organism to withstand months and years of anoxia. In between, there are numerous cases which have been incompletely investigated, in which survival continues for intermediate periods. One such case has recently been reported by Robin and coworkers. The experimental animals which were used in the investigation were the fresh-water turtles of the genus *Pseudemys*. *Pseudemys* can survive total immersion for as long as two weeks, which, even taking into account their ability to survive conditions which would normally be fatal to warm blooded animals, is a long time. During this time, they show a reduced sensitivity to cyanide in concentrations that might be expected to be fatal for normally active turtles. As one of the effects of cyanide is to inhibit electron transport, it seems reasonable to presume that the turtles switch over to a totally anaerobic metabolism. This is confirmed by a rise in the level of blood lactic acid during the experiment, and is corroborated by some earlier results obtained by another group with different turtle species, which showed that a specific inhibitor of glycolysis was fatal to submerged turtles in doses which they could survive under normal conditions.

As the same limitations with regard to brain and cardiac tissues ought to apply to turtles as well as to other vertebrates, lactic dehydrogenase from these organs was studied. There proved to be little difference between enzymes from the two sources as far as the H and M polypeptide chains were concerned. Although this work is not complete, it is suggested that the unusual properties of the dehydrogenases may be symptomatic of an important mechanism which permits survival for prolonged periods of anoxia.

4.5   Hibernation

Hibernation and aestivation are both responses on the part of the animal to an adverse season. Many animals react to adverse conditions by migration; a relatively simple process which serves to remove the animal from an environment which has suddenly proved hostile obviates the need for any other more complicated processes, although sometimes the mechanisms which make an organism capable of journeys of thousands of miles are themselves very complex. An alternative solution to physical withdrawal from environmental rigours is metabolic withdrawal, while remaining physically present. It is the essence both of hibernation, which refers to the reaction taking place in winter, and aestivation, which is a similar process occurring in summer.

Like all processes, the terms are subject to the differences of opinion of workers in the field, and, following considerable dissent over the precise nature of hibernation, the currently accepted concept does not completely coincide with the layman's view. For example, in spite of preconceptions about tortoises it is doubtful whether true hibernation is ever exhibited by groups other than mammals. Certainly, many reptiles inhabiting temperate environments exhibit a complete torpidity during the cold weather. They rapidly revive, however, on being warmed up, and just as rapidly revert to the torpid condition on cooling. It is not uncommon to see them emerge on warm days in winter, which is something that a true hibernator seldom does. Thus, in all but those groups which are capable of temperature regulation, and maintain a body temperature significantly above that of their environment, seasonal activity is directly dependent on the ambient temperature.

Only two groups have attained the ability to regulate body temperature by internal mechanisms, although many groups do so by behavioural mechanisms which involve avoiding or basking in direct sunlight. The two groups are the mammals and the birds. Even then, hibernation is a poor thing in birds by comparison with mammals. It is confined to some North American species—poorwills, swallows and swifts—which enter a state of torpidity which resembles hibernation in that the body temperature drops markedly. Mammals are, to all intents and purposes, to be considered the only vertebrate class that is capable of true hibernation.

Many hibernators accumulate fatty deposits in the Autumn in preparation for the cold weather. Among the fat deposits laid down are often stores of the so-called brown-fat. It is a rather special tissue, which is also frequently found in the new born young of many mammals, and also in adults of several non-hibernating species. The function of the brown fat has been much in dispute; in many hibernators, it is apparently capable of a very rapid metabolism which is divorced from the need to synthesize ATP. It is permanently uncoupled, and its oxidative processes are directed towards the production of heat, both during hibernation and during arousal from hibernation. In the hedgehog (*Erinaceus europaeus*), brown fat proved to be the warmest tissue in the animal when it was returning to activity in a warm environment; its temperature was almost 4°C above that of the heart. A similar situation occurs in the bat.

Brown fat is particularly rich in cytochromes, which to a great extent accounts for its characteristic colour. All the usual components of the electron transport system have been detected in it, and, in addition, two unusual components of the cytochrome b group. It seems that there are certainly alternative pathways of electron transport in this tissue, although it has not yet been possible to implicate the two new cytochromes. The most

4

likely alternative route of electron transfer is by way of a terminal oxidase involving, not a haemoprotein like cytochrome, but a flavoprotein. Such an oxidase would completely short circuit the energy producing portion of the electron transport system, and the energy of electron transfer would be dissipated as heat. This particular respiratory adaptation is almost certainly not the only reaction sequence in the tissue with a heat generating or thermogenic function. There are also the reactions involving the fats themselves.

The metabolism of the remainder of the animal during hibernation has not been the subject of nearly such intensive study as the brown fat. Thermogenesis by brown fat is an aerobic process; however, some recent work has indicated that anaerobic oxidative processes in other tissues may make a significant contribution to the heat gain of the animal. It is suggested that the body temperature would have to rise several degrees to a critical level of about $11°C$ before aerobic metabolism of carbohydrates accelerated markedly, and that prior to this, heat would have to be supplied from glycolytic activity, supplemented at later stages by heat generated in muscular movement.

There is also evidence that the phosphorylation efficiencies of tissues from hibernating and non-hibernating mammals differ at different temperatures. In cold-adapted rats and rabbits (animals which have been maintained for considerable periods of time in the cold) oxidative phosphorylation shows a degree of uncoupling, which does not happen in the hibernators. Conversely, the rate of oxidative phosphorylation in the cardiac muscle from rats, measured at $38°C$, was significantly higher than that from hibernating hamsters. Thus, while the same processes go on the tissues of both groups of animals, rat tissue requires a higher energy of activation than does hamster tissue. When this is combined with the actual increase in the concentration of enzymes during hibernation, it is obvious that we are dealing with a manifestation of one of the adaptations which permit the phenomenon of hibernation to take place.

The differing responses of enzymes from hibernators and non-hibernators implies a different composition and a different stability for these enzymes. Non-hibernators are adapted to function at high temperatures, and hibernators are adapted to the lower part of the range. Such differences could well be traced to the macromolecular structures of the enzymes concerned; it is an attractive hypothesis that, as the isoenzymes of lactic dehydrogenase are important in switching metabolism from its aerobic to its anaerobic phase, so isoenzymes may confer on the hibernators their special ability to survive cold and the torpidity of hibernation.

4.6 Diapause

Diapause is a phenomenon which reaches its greatest manifestation in insects, although it is not unlikely that it occurs in other arthropod groups, and may even occur in other invertebrates and vertebrates. It is not a physiological state which can easily be defined, and the word 'diapause' is a loose one which is interpreted in many ways depending on the inclination of the observer and the nature of the group of animals upon which he happens to work.

In essence, diapause is an interruption in the normal behaviour, activity or development of an organism which has its origin from within the organism itself. In this way, it can be separated from the process of hibernation which is brought on by the adverse winter conditions. Diapause may be triggered by some aspect of the external environment, but the triggering is followed by a complex series of physiological and biochemical adjustments which are inevitable, and dictated by the genetic structure of the animal.

Diapause, then, is an innate mechanism which ensures that the life of the animal is synchronized with its environment, and may be exhibited by developing eggs, by larval stages, by pupae or by adults. It may be triggered by temperature, the relative proportions of light and dark in the day, the supply and nature of food stuffs available, the density of population and many other factors. It persists until the appropriate stimulus indicates that the favourable moment for the resumption of activity has arrived.

One of its characteristics is that growth and other energy consuming processes are arrested. Energy requirements are reduced to a minimum, and the symptom of this state is a great reduction in respiration. During diapause, the animal becomes much less sensitive to chemicals which inhibit the respiratory processes. It was early discovered that carbon monooxide and cyanide had very little effect on some insects in diapause. As these substances are, in low concentrations, specific inhibitors of terminal electron transfer, either the conditions of diapause did not permit their access to the enzyme—which is unlikely as the inhibitors are small molecules—or some radical change had overtaken the respiratory chain during diapause.

The Cecropia moth, *Hyalophora cecropia*, has been extensively used for studies of cytochromes in insects, both during normal activity and during diapause. Three types of distribution of cytochromes are found in these moths. The first is found in the muscles of all stages of the life-cycle, and conforms to the classic pattern described in Chapter 2. In the non-muscular tissue of the larva and of the adult, however, a brand new component appears. It almost completely obscures the spectra of cytochromes b and c; it belongs to the b group of cytochromes and is designated cytochrome b_5. At one time it was considered a likely candidate for the terminal oxidase, replacing the oxygen dependent cytochrome oxidase, of the diminished respiratory activity of the diapausing moth, but later studies showed that it was similar to a cytochrome which is found in mammalian microsomes. Like its mammalian counterpart, insect cytochrome b_5 is not found in the mitochondria, and therefore probably has other functions than respiration.

The third pattern of cytochromes is found in the pupa of the moth during diapause.

At the onset of diapause, the classical cytochromes b and c disappear, and the concentrations of cytochrome a and cytochrome oxidase become vanishingly small, a fact which explains in great part the reduced sensitivity of the pupa to inhibitors. The extramitochondrial cytochrome also becomes less evident. When diapause ends, the cytochromes rapidly reappear.

In order to understand this, it must be explained that the developing egg is characterized by the possession of cytochrome b_5 and cytochrome a. This pattern does not change, even when the egg enters diapause, although the concentrations of the cytochromes may decrease, either due to breakdown of the old or failure to synthesize the new haemoprotein. The pattern is thus similar to that observed in the pupa during diapause, and it is thought that its re-emergence at this time is due to the breakdown of the larval cells which are then replaced by persistent embryonic cells which have retained the embryonic cytochromes. Thus, the modified cytochrome system is not necessarily a direct result of the condition of diapause, but rather due to a requirement for the processes of development.

The role of the ubiquitous cytochrome b_5 is not understood. It appears unlikely to have any function as a terminal oxidase, and may act in ion transport or protein synthesis. Even though the classical cytochromes are reduced to very low levels, their concentration is consistent with the observed respiratory requirements of the pupa—some two per cent of the non-diapausing level. The reduced effect of cyanide and carbon monoxide

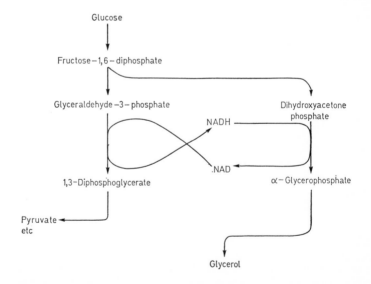

Fig. 4-2 The production of glycerol by dispausing insects.

is due to the fact that, although the concentrations of the cytochromes b and c are very small, so as to be rate limiting in electron transport, those of cytochrome a and cytochrome oxidase are considerably greater, even though they too are present in much lower concentrations. Thus even in the presence of the inhibitors, the small amount of the oxidase which remains uninhibited is still sufficient to cope with the electron transfer from cytochromes b and c.

From this it follows that anaerobic respiration is of great importance in diapausing insects. Apart from the more usual metabolic pathways, one leading to the formation of glycerol assumes considerable importance. In one case, the concentration of the end product reaches such high proportions that it has been postulated that it might act as an anti-freeze, and serve to protect tissues from the triturating effects of ice crystal formation during exposure to low temperatures.

During the formation of glycerol, reduced pyridine nucleotides are re-oxidized; thus glycerol represents an oxygen debt which may subsequently have to be repaid, but which permits the synthesis of ATP (Fig. 4–2).

5.1 Introduction

This particular heterogeneous group of animals has been chosen for detailed consideration merely because more is known about them than any other group of ostensible anaerobes of a higher organization than bacteria. Intestinal helminths exemplify the most elegant of known solutions to the general problem of doing without oxygen, in spite of the fact that the study of parasites poses special problems; all too often, insufficient material is available for experiments, and elaborate and expensive culturing techniques are often required.

Once obtained, the material may be contaminated, perhaps by bacteria from the gut, or by tissues from the host itself. There is an ever present suspicion that the researcher may be investigating the host and its symbionts rather than the parasite. Of necessity, the experiments must be carried out in *in vitro* systems which involve removing the parasite from the host. A parasite thus divorced from its environment is like a fish out of water; it behaves atypically out of its true biological context. Such is the delicate and intimate balance of the host-parasite relationship that it is doubtful whether one can achieve more than the coarsest approximation of its ramifications with any great validity. The host provides many important physiological and biochemical essentials that the parasite lacks; this, after all, is the stuff of parasitism and to study the parasite in their absence is fraught with danger and misconception because to live *in* an intestine is almost like having an intestine of your own. If this is not enough, by the time the experimenter has made his various cellular and sub-cellular preparations, the validity of the experiment is even more questionable. It is only because much work with mammals has demonstrated the effectiveness of this particular experimental approach that the work has any value at all. After all, one has to start somewhere.

The concepts, aerobic or anaerobic, as applied to parasites, need careful examination. It is doubtful whether any of the parasitic helminths can be made to conform entirely with either category, although some of the parasitic protozoa may be true anaerobes. The nature of the environment of the parasite is such that there will almost always be some oxygen present, even if it is only in vanishingly small quantities. As all organisms are, to speak teleologically, metabolic opportunists, if a resource is available and is useful, then it will be used. Its use need not be confined to respiration alone, for there are many other processes that require oxygen. The parasites assume a chamaeleon-like physiological quality—the type of their metabolism whether aerobic or anaerobic is fitted to the prevailing environmental condition. They must therefore possess some mechanism which will enable them to detect and to react to a change in that environment; the precise nature of this mechanism is one that still mystifies parasitologists.

The foregoing paragraph is not meant to imply that parasites are facultative anaerobes, that there are two mutually exclusive alternatives—to use oxygen or not to use it—one of which is turned on at a given time to be replaced by the other when the environment changes. Some parasites may indeed exhibit this pattern, but more usually the inaccuracy of the methods of study do not permit the investigator to perceive that differences are differences of degree and are not qualitative. According to this reasoning, the facultative anaerobe is at one end of the spectrum and the obligate aerobe is at the other, but they differ from one another only in the relative conspicuousness of their aerobic and anaerobic modes.

5.2 Metabolic pathways in parasites

Although the tricarboxylic acid does not usually function in the absence of oxygen, the individual reactions of which it is composed, and which are not intrinsically dependent on the presence of oxygen, may still occur and may be of fundamental importance. Thus, in many of the parasitic protozoa, of which the blood-parasitic trypanosomes may be cited as an example, the dehydrogenase enzymes of the cycle have been detected in the most anaerobic species. Similarly, in intestinal helminths, a complete tricarboxylic acid cycle, albeit with greatly diminished activity, has been detected in the tape-worms, *Echinococcus* and *Moniezia*, in the round-worm *Ascaris*, and in the liver-fluke, *Fasciola hepatica*, which, while it is not a gut parasite, is a representative of a group in which this way of life predominates.

The use to which this pathway is put by the parasitic helminths differs greatly from the orthodox and accepted function. Instead of participating in the oxidation of pyruvic acid to carbon dioxide and water, a different sequence of reactions occurs. Pyruvic acid is carboxylated to yield either malic or oxaloacetic acids. The product is then converted to succinic acid by a reversal of the malic dehydrogenase, fumarase and succinic dehydrogenase reactions of the tricarboxylic acid cycle (Fig. 5–1). The process is very similar to that described in bacteria some forty years ago, and was later detected in *Ascaris* by Bueding and coworkers. This early observation has since been extended to several cestodes and trematodes.

The fate of the succinic acid so produced is of considerable importance. It is possible to draw parallels with the fate of lactic acid produced by glycolysis. In the tape-worm *Moniezia expansa*, succinate accumulates in the medium in which the worm is maintained. It is excreted. The tape-worm may thus be considered to have built up an oxygen debt which it is never called upon to discharge; it merely removes the oxygen equivalent

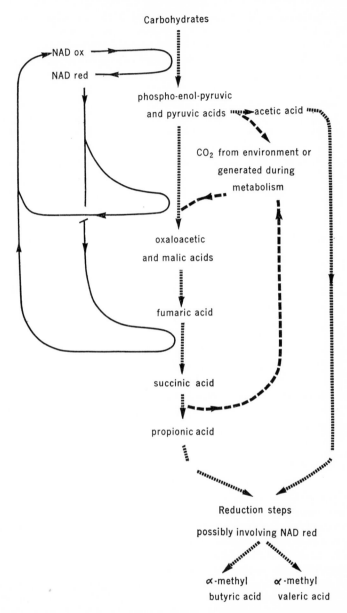

Fig. 5–1 The fixation of carbon dioxide, the reoxidation of NAD and the excretion of acids by parasitic helminths. The formation of propionic acid and its subsequent condensation with acetic acid to yield methyl butyric and valeric acids has only been demonstrated in *Ascaris*, the pig round-worm.

from within itself. In *Ascaris*, a very different situation obtains. Some, a small proportion only, of the succinate is excreted. The remainder undergoes a series of decarboxylation and reduction reactions which yield a whole series of acids (Fig. 5–1). Once again the oxygen debt is not repaid as the acids are excreted.

The functions of these additional pathways are twofold. As in the case of lactic acid production, they effectively reduce the concentration of pyruvic acid formed by the anaerobic degradation of carbohydrates, thus removing the possibility that ATP producing mechanisms are subject to product inhibition. They also permit the reoxidation of reduced cofactors, so that the latter are once again able to participate in the anaerobic energy producing pathways.

It must be clearly understood that this interpretation is a simplification. Lactic acid itself is excreted by many parasites, and its significance can be explained in the normal way. Other parasites produce other acids, and a given parasite may change the nature of its acid excretion if the environment varies; it seems likely however that the same general principles apply. Considerable work is currently in progress in this field, and in spite of the difficulties inherent in the study, it is probable that the near future will provide us with a clearer understanding of metabolic regulation in parasites.

5.3   Electron transport in parasites

It is not surprising, in view of the diverse methods adopted by parasites to overcome the problem of life in the absence of a plentiful supply of oxygen, that respiratory electron transport systems bear only a superficial similarity to that of the mammals. It is a confused area of knowledge. In trypanosomes, for example, cytochromes a and b have been identified, but not c. Cytochrome oxidase has been variously reported to be present and absent in the same species! Much of the confusion derives from the use of blood-stream forms or cultured forms of the trypanosomes; the latter resemble the forms found in the insect host rather than the mammalian one. Thus, although investigators are working with the same species of protozoan, the two forms may be considered to be different physiological entities. This illustrates rather nicely the problems biochemists encounter when they investigate the metabolism of parasites which require two or three different species of host to complete their life-cycle.

It is clear that the parasite must be adapted to each host. It could achieve this by possessing completely separate sets of enzymes, and in a given host, only the appropriate ones function. Alternatively, adaptation to a variety of hosts could be obtained by a mechanism which permitted only the sequential expression of the parasite's capability for producing enzymes. The most likely level for this to work would be at the genetic one, the activity of the genes being initiated by the appropriate stimulus from the host at the appropriate time. The problem of the switch from one type of metabolism to another when the parasite changes hosts will be considered briefly in the following section.

Somewhat more is known about the parasitic helminths. The first worm to be studied from this point of view was *Ascaris*. One group of workers found cytochrome oxidase, dehydrogenases and a capacity for the re-oxidation of cytochrome c in muscle. This suggested that a cytochrome

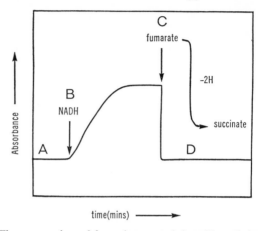

Fig. 5–2 The conversion of fumaric to succinic acid, and the involvement of cytochrome in this reaction in parasitic worms. The measurements are made at the wavelength of greatest absorption by cytochrome. The cytochrome remains in the oxidized condition (A) until NADH is added (B) when it rapidly becomes reduced, with an increase in absorbance. At equilibrium, fumaric acid is added (C). The cytochrome becomes reoxidized; at the same time, fumaric is converted to succinic acid (D).

system was of some importance in this animal, and subsequent studies with drugs supported the view. A brand new cytochrome was also detected in the helminth.

At the same time, however, another group of workers demonstrated that respiration and the formation of succinate from fumarate continued without the participation of a cytochrome system. Terminal oxidation in this reaction was mediated by a flavoprotein.

In tape worms, *Moniezia expansa* has been investigated in some detail. This parasite was found to have a branched respiratory chain. The branch occurred at a point between the flavoprotein and the cytochrome components of the respiratory chain. One branch led to an orthodox cytochrome system, similar to that found in mammals. It was present in such small quantities that it was at first overlooked because it was masked by a second component. The latter contained one or more new cytochromes, the terminal one of which had a spectrum similar to the new one which had previously been found in *Ascaris*. The remarkable thing about this cytochrome was that, *in vitro*, it became reduced when the electron transport pathway was made to oxidize NADH. It stayed reduced in the presence of oxygen. However, when fumaric acid was added to the incubation medium, the cytochrome became reoxidized, and the fumarate was reduced to succinate.

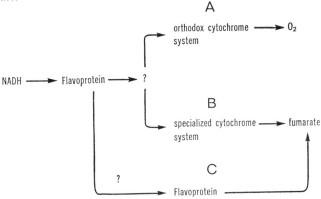

Fig. 5–3 Cytochrome systems in parasitic worms. These organisms apparently possess a branched chain system. One branch leads to an orthodox electron transfer path (A), the other to a specialized system in which fumaric acid acts as an electron acceptor (either B or C).

Here, then, was a system in which fumaric acid apparently substituted for oxygen as the ultimate electron acceptor in a cytochrome system. A similar process of reversed electron transfer had already been observed in mammalian mitochondria under experimental conditions, but in the helminth preparation it appeared to be a major pathway. Investigations of other intestinal helminths suggest that the pathway is widespread; similar cytochromes have been detected in representatives of the other parasitic groups. In the liver fluke, preliminary accounts indicate that the conversion of fumarate to succinate may be accompanied by a net synthesis of ATP, although this awaits verification.

There are objections to the above hypothesis. For example, there is a cytochrome of the endoplasmic reticulum of mammals which has rather similar properties to the terminal cytochrome in the proposed parasitic pathway. As the preparation of mitochondria from parasites has by no means reached the degree of sophistication of the mammalian studies, it is not impossible that the new cytochrome may derive from endoplasmic reticulum and not from mitochondria.

5.4   The switch mechanism

One of the problems already hinted at in this chapter is the plight of a parasite which has to adapt to more than one host in its life cycle. The

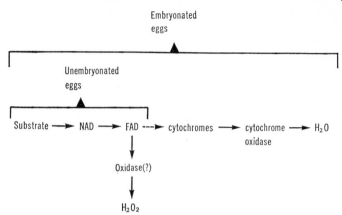

Fig. 5-4 The switch mechanism in *Ascaris* eggs. Embryonation and the extension of the cytochrome system to include cytochrome oxidase occur simultaneously.

factors responsible for the adaptive switch are only just beginning to be unravelled. For example, it is known that the stimulus which encourages the encysted cercaria—an immature form of the liver fluke—to leave its cyst, which it has secreted around itself after emerging from its snail host, is the presence of reducing conditions in the gut of the mammalian host. Whether there are any biochemical preparations in anticipation of the ingestion by the mammalian host is not yet known. In the same way, the sloughing of the cuticle of the developing nematode parasite is brought about as a response to a definite chemical stimulus.

The most complete study of the switch to date has been carried out on *Ascaris* eggs. It was found that unembryonated eggs of *Ascaris* lacked cytochromes and their pattern of metabolism generally resembled that of the adult, as they converted fumaric acid to succinic by a pathway involving flavoproteins. These eggs require to be exposed to oxygen before the embryos develop. In embryonated—infective, that is—eggs, there is a full cytochrome system. The eggs are ingested and develop in the gut of the mammalian host; they switch back to the fumaric acid-succinic acid system. The conclusions drawn from these experiments are that cytochrome oxidase activity is included as a constitutive part of the enzyme armoury of all stages of the worm. The capacity for synthesizing cytochrome oxidase does not suddenly appear—it is there all the time. Only certain conditions, however, can call forth the expression of this genetic potential, and it appears that oxygen, as is the case in many yeasts, is the stimulus required. However, this must be modified by other factors because, as far as is known, exposing the adult to oxygen does not result in the formation of detectable quantities of cytochrome oxidase. Timing, the exact stage of the life history, and host stimulus are also of paramount importance.

Conclusions

It is obviously impossible in a book of this size to cover more than a very small portion of a whole wealth of literature. Much of the information it contains is enshrined as fact; a great deal more has yet to receive this accolade. Many of the conclusions described in the present work are derived from the latter; many of the observations are contentious, and in these areas work is being carried out with an intensity which means that what has been accepted today is obsolete tomorrow.

Within these limitations, a few tentative conclusions may be drawn. There is a comforting uniformity to life. Whatever the differences in external morphology, all animals are subject to the same basic restrictions, because they must all obey the same scientific principles. Their selection of habit imposes further restrictions, but adaptation to an environment must be made with whatever internal resources the organism has at its disposal. The first thing that determines the success or failure of an animal in a particular environment is its genetic potential. The expression of its genetic potential is manifested through the manipulation of complex molecules such as proteins. A protein, however, is subject to the same vagaries of fortune, and obeys the same laws whether it is produced by an amoeba or an elephant. It often performs the same function in both, as there are only a limited number of ways of doing things efficiently.

The fact that there is only a limited number of ways of doing things is of fundamental importance in evolution, as it results in biological conservatism. Once an efficient mechanism appears, it will be selected, and its selection will continue until there is a radical change in the environment which reduces its efficiency. Even then it may not be superseded as there may not be a sufficiently efficient and functional alternative.

The brand new solution to a biological problem, the innovation in evolution is something which must happen very rarely indeed, if at all. Evolution does not proceed by fits and starts; it is a continuous process of which the unit is the population. In any given population there is a usually normal distribution of variation. All dogs have the general property of dogness which does not require definition. One of the properties which go to make up dogness is the possession of a tail. Some dogs have long tails, others have short ones, and in between there is every sort of length.

The initiating fact of evolution does not come from within the animal, but it is imposed on the animal by the environment. Recent evolutionary theory suggests that evolutionary change is subsequent to a behavioural change in an animal. For example, the animals at the periphery (and it does not have to be a geographical periphery) of a population are pushed by pressures from within the population into an environment which departs from the ideal for that species at that point in time. In this less than perfect environment, the animals either adapt or succumb. Those that survive obviously exhibited behavioural and somatic characteristics which permitted their survival, and selection followed.

Now, if the hypothetical dogs occupied an environment in which tails were of no great advantage, but some peripheral dogs occasionally moved into environments where a selection pressure was set up for longer tails, then a breed of dogs would appear which were endowed with long tails. Dogs, however, are still recognizably dogs, and tails are still more recognizably tails. The disinterested observer would note a greater similarity between the tails than between the dogs that bore them. And the same may be said for their respiratory metabolisms.

Parasitic protozoa and helminths, insects, other arthropods and vertebrates all tend to do certain fundamental things in the same way. Haemoproteins are useful molecules because of their capacity for binding small molecules, and their relatively easy transitions from the reduced to the oxidized state and vice versa. The first property made them suitable for use as transporting molecules, for respiratory gases, for small molecules in complex synthetic reactions, and for ions. Their capacity for electron transport has resulted in their incorporation with other molecules into complex respiratory chains. Their degree of efficiency is such that there is no real alternative to their use. If the animal finds itself in an environment which detracts from the efficiency of its respiratory system, it has the alternatives of removing itself from that environment, or making do with what it already has. The latter involves making changes in the components of the system within the framework of the principle which is of proven efficiency.

Anaerobiosis as a way of life appears to be totally feasible, even to organisms which in the evolutionary past have committed themselves to the aerobic way of life. In hibernation, diapause, and intestinal parasitism there is a great dependence on the presumably more archaic pathway of glycolysis. The dependence is imposed, in the case of the hibernator, by the necessity to survive low temperatures which render the activity of the cytochrome system less efficient; in the case of the insect, by the ablation for the period of diapause of the majority of those cytochromes which are responsible for respiration; and in the case of the parasites, by environmental limitations.

It is probably no coincidence that in each of the three cases one or more cytochromes of the b group are implicated. It is a pity that so little is known about their functions. In the brown fat of the hibernating mammal, the function of the cytochrome b is patently unknown; in the insect it was once thought to function as the terminal oxidase, although this has now been shown to be untrue; in the parasite it may conceivably act as the terminal oxidase. It is also interesting to note that in all three cases, a flavoprotein oxidase system has been described, which by-passes the cytochrome system.

In trying to make any general statements on the basis of this work, it must be borne in mind that very few species have been studied. Perhaps the most complete area is that occupied by the parasites. Most intestinal parasites react in the same way to their environments; carbon dioxide fixation and the conversion of fumaric acid to succinic loom large in their metabolisms. Fumaric acid or molecules like it apparently substitute for oxygen in the cytochrome system. The source of the acceptor molecule is internal, so that the parasite is freed from one, at least, of the restrictions of its environment. It is a mechanism which is adopted by an animal which can afford to be 'wasteful'; it is bathed in a sea of nutrients, and therefore to excrete substances which could be oxidized further is not a serious drain on its economy. Although these pathways have the advantage of effecting the reoxidation of reduced cofactors, the advantage would be much greater if accompanied by a net synthesis of ATP.

There is a possibility that this pathway is related directly to the parasitic habit. Unfortunately, far too few examples of free-living representatives of the groups have been studied, and those that have may be specialized and hence atypical. However, in some protozoa, including amoeba, alternative pathways of electron transport are present, and one free-living flatworm and one free-living nematode are reported to have a cytochrome similar to that found in parasites. It seems likely, therefore, that the metabolic modifications encountered in the respiratory mechanisms of parasites are not a direct result of the adoption of the parasitic mode of life. Instead, it seems more probable that those groups, whose ancestors were already adapted to life in situations where constant high oxygen tensions could not be relied on, were already partly equipped for survival in the intestine. It was a ready-made adaptation when they made the transition from ecto- to endoparasitism. The intestine is, after all, only a special case of an oxygen deficient environment. Many other animals show similar modifications to oxygen deficiency—for example, some bivalve molluscs excrete succinic acid into their environments. The success of the parasites must therefore be due, in part at least, to their derivation from groups already adapted to the oxygen-less life, and, in part, to their ability to evolve adequate protection mechanisms against the depredations of the host biochemistry. The fact that the first problem was already solved must have given them an immense selective advantage.

Short term solutions to the problems of life in the absence of oxygen have also been shown to be possible, and are based on essentially the same mechanism. The switching off of the cytochrome system and the dependence on glycolysis is almost ubiquitous. Lactic dehydrogenase is at least one important switch. The principle of the oxygen debt is also universal— the only difference is the coin in which it is repaid.

The examples of conservatism mentioned here are by no means unique; it is certain that it extends to all biochemical systems. A law of parsimony operates in nature, but all it really says is that the building blocks are essentially identical. True variation stems from the shape into which they are pressed.

Further Reading

BARKER, GEOFFREY R. (1968). *Understanding the Chemistry of the Cell* (Studies in Biology 13). Edward Arnold, London.

BENNETT THOMAS P. and FRIEDEN, EARL (1966). *Modern Topics in Biochemistry —The Structure and Function of Biological Molecules*. Macmillan, London.

BRYANT, C. (1970). Electron Transport in Parasitic Helminths and Protozoa. *Adv. in Parasit.*, **8**, p. 139. Academic Press, London and New York.

GILMOUR, DARCY (1961). *The Biochemistry of Insects*. Academic Press, London and New York.

LEHNINGER, ALBERT L. (1965). *Bioenergetics*. Benjamin, New York.

MOROWITZ, HAROLD J. (1963). *Life and the Physical Sciences—Introduction to Biophysics*. Holt, Rinehart and Winston, New York and London.

ROODYN, D. B. and WILKIE, D. (1968). *The Biogenesis of Mitochondria*. Methuen, London.

SCHMIDT-NIELSEN, KNUT (1964). *Animal Physiology* (Foundations of Modern Biology), Prentice-Hall. London.

SPEAKMAN, J. D. (1966). *Molecules*. McGraw-Hill, Maidenhead.

WILLIAMS, ROGER J. (1963). *Biochemical Individuality*. Wiley, New York and Chichester.